Birth Trauma

Birth Trauma

A guide for you, your friends and family to coping with post-traumatic stress disorder following birth

Kim Thomas

NELL JAMES PUBLISHERS

Published by Nell James Publishers
www.nelljames.co.uk
info@nelljames.co.uk

British Library Cataloguing-in-Publication Data
A catalogue record for this book is available from the British Library.

ISBN 978-0-9567024-7-0

First published 2013.

The Publisher has no responsibility for the persistence or accuracy of URLs for external or any third-party internet websites referred to in this book, and does not guarantee that any content on such websites is, or will remain, accurate or appropriate.

Note: The advice and information included in this book is published in good faith. However, the Publisher and author assume no responsibility or liability for any loss, injury or expense incurred as a result of relying on the information stated. Please check with the relevant persons and authorities regarding any legal and medical issues.

Printed in Great Britain.

Contents

Introduction

In August 2012, a national newspaper ran a moving account of women who had suffered post-traumatic stress disorder (PTSD) after giving birth.[1] One woman, Kelly, described how her baby was born 'limp and blue after the cord became wrapped around his neck'. The midwife then took the baby from the room, and Kelly, convinced the baby had died, started haemorrhaging from a tear she'd experienced while giving birth. Although the baby was fine, Kelly suffered frequent nightmares and flashbacks to the birth until she received treatment.

On the newspaper's website, the article attracted numerous comments. Some, including ones from women who had had similar experiences, were sympathetic, but others insisted that in the past women 'just got on with it' or that the symptoms described were just a product of the 'blame culture'. Several said that it was wrong to compare the experience of giving birth with the experience of fighting a war, one of the most well-known causes of PTSD.

The comments demonstrate that many people still have a poor understanding of what PTSD is and what causes it. Perhaps it is not surprising that many still associate it with war, because the earliest recorded accounts of PTSD – or shell shock as it was then known – come from men returning from World War I. Many experienced nightmares and vivid flashbacks that would suddenly appear in their mind as if from nowhere. One infantry captain described how, in a flashback, 'the face of a Boche that I have bayoneted comes sharply into view.'[2] Some men found that they could no longer eat or sleep properly.

It wasn't until the late 1970s that the term 'shell shock', which was believed originally to be the result of physical injury to the nerves, was replaced by 'post traumatic stress disorder' (PTSD) and recognised as a psychiatric disorder. Doctors soon came to realise that PTSD wasn't confined to soldiers, but could happen to anyone who had been through a violent and frightening experience, such as a physical assault, a car accident or a terrorist attack. PTSD occurs when someone has believed their own life or someone else's to be under threat, or when they have witnessed a terrible event, such as another person's death.

There are good reasons why a woman who has suffered a difficult birth might be susceptible to PTSD. Although it is rare in modern developed countries for women to die in childbirth, things can still go wrong, and a woman who has lost a lot of blood, for example, may easily feel her life is in danger. And the fear of losing a baby is all too real: more than 4,000 babies are stillborn in the UK every year. Other babies are born with disabilities, such as cerebral palsy, which can be caused by a lack of oxygen during the birth, or Erb's palsy, a paralysis to the arm, shoulder or hand, often caused when the baby is stuck in the birth canal and too much force is applied when trying to pull the baby out. Women whose babies have died or been damaged by the birth process can suffer from PTSD, as can women who have simply feared that their babies would die.

Although the possibility that the experience of a traumatic childbirth could lead to PTSD wasn't recognised until the 1980s, Jean Robinson, president of the Alliance for Improvement in Maternity Services (AIMS), says she became aware of it 10 years earlier. In the 1970s, when she was chair of the Patients Association, she received hundreds of letters from women describing symptoms of trauma:

> 'What many of the women were describing was like the shell shock I had read about in the histories of the First World War. But those mothers were in limbo: they had a condition which officially did not exist.'[3]

The early 1970s, she writes, is a time when many women found the experience of giving birth traumatic, because of the new enthusiasm among obstetricians for inducing 'overdue' women (who in many cases may not really have been overdue) by giving them synthetic hormones that caused intense, painful contractions without softening the cervix in readiness for the baby to pass through. Childbirth for these women was often agonising.

Jean Robinson came to realise, however, that PTSD wasn't unique to women who had experienced obstetric intervention. Many women who had experienced a difficult birth, particularly if they felt the attendant doctors or midwives had been unsympathetic, also went on to develop trauma symptoms:

> 'In our tiny office at the Patients Association I had been dealing with hundreds of complaints about every kind of medical care, but the childbirth letters stood out. It was their vividness and the intensity of memories described which made me realise something was happening.'[4]

Many of those letters came not just from mothers but from grandmothers whose memories of a difficult childbirth had stayed with them all their lives. If the terms 'PTSD' and 'birth trauma' are relatively new, the experience of them is certainly not.

How this book can help
Although doctors now recognise that the experience of giving birth can give rise to PTSD, awareness is still limited. Some women who experience PTSD symptoms do not realise what is happening to them, and they may be misdiagnosed by their GP as suffering from postnatal depression (PND). More than half of women with PTSD do also suffer from PND, making diagnosis complicated. Similarly, there is still a lot we don't know about PTSD after giving birth: researchers have only started working on the area in the past 20 years, often using small-scale studies, and there are large gaps in our knowledge. We still don't know, for example, why some women who have had traumatic birth experiences go on to develop PTSD while others don't.

Women who have suffered PTSD after giving birth may feel isolated. It can feel as if there is no-one to turn to, and that partners, family and friends expect them to 'move on'. My aim in writing this book is to help women who have suffered PTSD after giving birth to find the support they need. Although it is mostly aimed at the women themselves, I also hope that partners, families and friends of sufferers will find it helpful, and that health professionals will also gain some insight into the experiences of women who have undergone a traumatic birth.

The book uses real-life examples of women who have suffered either full-blown PTSD or some trauma symptoms after giving birth. Despite their terrible experiences, all the women who spoke to me have made full or partial recoveries. I hope this book will help to show that, however frightening the experience of PTSD is at the time, it is possible with the right support to recover and lead a normal life.

The book has six chapters in total, covering the following issues:

Chapter 1: What is birth trauma? This looks at the causes of birth trauma, the criteria for diagnosing it and some of the typical symptoms.

Chapter 2: You and your baby. Women who have experienced birth trauma often find it difficult to bond with their baby. The chapter looks at how mothers' relationship with their baby is affected by birth trauma and what can be done to help establish that bond.

Chapter 3: Partners, family and friends. Birth trauma can damage the relationship between a woman and those close to her, particularly her partner, who may also be traumatised or may find it difficult to understand what she's going through. This chapter looks at how relationships change in the wake of birth trauma.

Chapter 4: Treatment and recovery. Two therapies have been found to be particularly effective in treating PTSD, and this chapter describes them in detail, as well as looking at other treatments you may find useful.

Chapter 5: Taking action. In extreme cases, such as ones where the mother or baby have been injured during the birth, it may be advisable to take legal action against the hospital trust.

This chapter explains how to do that and looks at other options, such as complaining to the hospital. It also looks at what you can do to campaign for change in maternity care.

Chapter 6: Getting better. Although birth trauma can feel like an overwhelming experience when you're going through it, women can and do recover from it, and some even go on to have another baby. This chapter looks at the experiences of women who have come through the other side and at what helped them.

At the end, you will find an appendix containing a list of useful website addresses to help you find therapists and support groups, as well as a glossary defining terms relating to birth trauma.

Terminology

The Birth Trauma Association uses the term 'birth trauma' to describe the experience of PTSD or PTSD symptoms after birth. (It is possible to have some of the symptoms of PTSD without meeting all the requirements for a formal diagnosis of PTSD.) Following their example, I have chosen to use the term 'birth trauma', occasionally using 'PTSD' where the context demands it.

Case histories

Throughout this book, I use the examples of real women who have experienced birth trauma. In all, the stories of 13 women are included here. I found them through a mix of places, including Mumsnet, Netmums, NCT and the Birth Trauma Association's Facebook page. Some spoke to me at length on the phone, while a few wrote their experiences down. I also use the experience of two of the women's husbands in chapter 3.

Some people were happy for me to use their real names, while others asked for pseudonyms to be used. Two of the interviewees, Nina and Jon, wanted to make clear that their real names were used, because, as Nina puts it, 'We gave a true account of our experience to try and help others. It is our experience and we are proud to claim ownership of it.' I am pleased to be able to do that, and hope that their example helps other people to be open about their experience of birth trauma.

Acknowledgements

I am extremely grateful to the 13 women and two men who willingly shared their stories with me. For several of the women, talking about the experience took a lot of courage and in some cases it was the first time they had spoken in any detail about what had happened.

I would also like to thank the numerous experts who kindly gave their time to be interviewed for the book and, in some cases, reviewed chapters for me. Your help was invaluable.

Many thanks, too, to Lynn Balmforth of NCT, who kindly helped me to source scholarly articles and made my job much easier.

Finally, I couldn't have written this book without the help of Maureen Treadwell of the Birth Trauma Association, who not only spoke to me for the book, but allowed me to use the Association's Facebook group to find women willing to share their experiences.

Chapter 1: What is birth trauma?

Emma gave birth after a long and exhausting labour. She'd been given a drip of Syntocinon, a synthetic hormone, to speed up labour, and an epidural to remove the pain. After the baby was born, she had difficulty pushing the placenta out. When it was finally delivered, Emma felt the mood in the room change as it suddenly filled up with people:

> 'They were all looking in the bucket where the placenta was. And I kept saying, "Something's wrong, something's wrong", and they were all muttering, and saying, "It's fine, it's fine, it's fine", and I just knew that something was wrong.'

Emma describes what happened next:

> 'There were four or five people in the room, and the consultant walked in. I had my feet up in stirrups and she didn't acknowledge me, I didn't really know who she was. I now know that what she did was a manual removal of the placenta, which was the most painful thing I've experienced to this day. I don't think I'll ever get over the shock of it. I remember as it was happening, I could see her hand through my stomach moving around and the force of her doing it – I thought was going to push me off the end of the bed. And I remember looking at my husband, and he was cradling our newborn baby, and looking at the wall so he couldn't see, and then I thought, "Things are bad".'

At this point, the midwife tried to persuade the consultant obstetrician to stop, but she carried on. Then things got worse:

'My husband said at this point the blood started shooting out. He said it was hitting the walls opposite, and it was like something from a horror film. He said the consultant looked at me, and the first time she acknowledged me, she said, "You need to come to theatre now, we need to give you some stitches," and walked out the room.'

As well as experiencing huge blood loss, Emma suffered a third degree tear, which is a tear extending from the vaginal wall and perineum to the anal sphincter. She was in hospital for five days, during which time she was given numerous drugs including antibiotics, morphine and codeine, and had a catheter attached to her.

It took a long time for Emma to recover physically from her experience. But she was left with deep and lasting emotional scars too. Although she didn't feel depressed, she couldn't listen to or watch anything relating to pregnancy or birth because it would induce feelings of panic in her. She felt enormous guilt for letting her baby down, because she wasn't well enough to look after her properly in the first three months of her life. Looking back on the birth, she says, 'In some ways it didn't feel real but in other ways it felt like I was reliving it and reliving it every minute of the day in my head.'

Emma was suffering from post-traumatic stress disorder (PTSD), a condition that occurs when, having experienced a terrible event, the person remains in psychological shock: they can't move on emotionally from the event.

What is PTSD?

The realisation amongst the medical profession that experiencing or witnessing a terrible event could cause a particular set of symptoms originated during the First World War, when soldiers returning from the war displayed symptoms such as flashbacks. Initially, the condition was known as 'shell shock' or 'battle fatigue'. Awareness of the condition increased after soldiers began returning from the Vietnam War with trauma symptoms. At the same time, psychologists were beginning to recognise that other victims of trauma, such as those who'd been raped or physically assaulted, displayed similar symptoms. In 1980, the term 'post-traumatic stress disorder' appeared in the third edition of the Diagnostic and Statistical Manual of Mental Disorders (DSM), the standard reference work used by psychiatrists in the United States and elsewhere.

As more research was carried out on PTSD sufferers, it was found that some traumatic experiences are more likely to lead to PTSD than others. People are more likely to develop PTSD after a man-made trauma, such as a terrorist attack, for example, than after a natural disaster, such as an earthquake.

In the 1980s, psychologists gradually began to identify the condition in women who'd given birth, though little research into the subject was done until the late 1990s. Even now, most of the research into PTSD after birth has involved small-scale studies rather than larger surveys. It means that what we know about PTSD after birth is still limited and tentative.

The onset of PTSD symptoms after giving birth is now frequently referred to as 'birth trauma'. As well as being a useful term, it avoids the implication that there is something 'disordered' about women's reactions to a frightening and sometimes life-threatening experience. As two psychologists who have written about birth trauma say:

> 'Theirs is, we would argue, a normal reaction to an extremely upsetting and horrific event.'[1]

How seriously should we take birth trauma?

Women who suffer from birth trauma often find that health professionals – as well as friends and relatives – have a poor understanding of the condition. Yet for women who undergo it, it is a frightening and debilitating experience. It can last for years, and can have a severe impact on their relationship with their baby and their partner, as well as on their ability to lead a normal life.

Although the maternal mortality rate in this country is low, suicide is one of the leading indirect causes.[2] (The maternal mortality rate refers to the numbers of women who die during pregnancy, during birth or within 42 days from the end of the pregnancy, from a cause relating to the pregnancy or birth. The reports on maternal mortality distinguish between deaths caused directly by the pregnancy or birth, such as infection, and deaths caused indirectly by the pregnancy or birth, such as heart problems or suicide.)

While it is well-known that postnatal depression (PND) can lead some women to commit suicide, some women with birth trauma also report suicidal feelings. We don't know how many maternal suicides are the result of birth trauma, but we need to be aware that the consequences of leaving birth trauma untreated are potentially serious.

Diagnosing birth trauma

When health professionals diagnose PTSD after birth, they use the same criteria that are used for diagnosing PTSD in other situations. These criteria are very precise – people who only meet some of the criteria are not said to be suffering from PTSD.

PTSD cannot be diagnosed in the first month following a trauma, as many people suffer symptoms in the initial aftermath of a trauma that disappear quite quickly. So to receive a diagnosis of PTSD, you have to have experienced the symptoms for at least a month.

There are two main sets of diagnostic criteria for PTSD, and they are outlined in manuals called ICD10, which is the World Health Organisation's classification of mental health disorders, and DSM. Neither of these distinguishes between birth trauma and other forms of PTSD. The two sets of criteria are very similar, but the most commonly used are the ones outlined in

DSM. (The ICD 10 diagnostic criteria are on the Department of Work and Pensions website.[3])

DSM

The DSM is the American Psychiatric Society's classification of mental health disorders – essentially the bible of the psychiatric profession. The fifth edition (DSM-5) was published in May 2013.

The classification of PTSD in DSM-5 states that the patient has to have been exposed to an 'extreme traumatic stressor' (usually involving death or injury) and the patient's response is characterised by one or more of four features: re-experiencing, avoidance, negative cognitions and mood, and arousal. It can only be diagnosed if the symptoms have been present for at least a month.[4]

Dr Susan Ayers, a psychologist and expert on birth trauma, summarises the currently used diagnostic criteria like this:

> 'At the moment in order to have a diagnosis of PTSD, you have to have been through an event in which you thought your own life, or that of somebody very important to you, was threatened, or their physical integrity was threatened, and then you need to respond with intense fear, helplessness or horror.'

Why do people suffer from PTSD?

Scientists are gradually coming to the conclusion that PTSD is caused by the failure of the brain to process memories in the normal way, so that a trauma that happened in the past still feels very real and present. One plausible explanation for how this happens is that, during a frightening situation, the body floods with the stress hormones adrenaline and cortisol, which disrupt the functioning of the hippocampus, a part of our brain responsible for memory processing and consolidation.

Because of the overwhelming emotions that we experience during a traumatic event, we don't process and remember the event in the same way that we process and remember normal events. As a result, we end up with a 'trauma memory', which has different qualities from our other every-day-life memories. Because the 'trauma memory' is not processed, it gets triggered very easily by situations that bear some resemblance to the original trauma, and our brain is tricked into thinking that the traumatic event is happening all over again. Our body then reacts in the same way as it did during the trauma, and we feel as if we are living through the event again in the here and now.

What causes birth trauma?

Birth trauma arises as the result of a frightening or upsetting experience during birth. To receive a formal diagnosis of PTSD, there has to have been a point during the labour where the mother feared that her own life or that of her baby was at risk.

Of the 13 women I spoke to for this book, for example, five had suffered postpartum haemorrhage. This refers to a loss of 500ml or more of blood after giving birth, and is the biggest cause of maternal death worldwide, accounting for 25% of deaths. It usually happens either because the placenta has been retained, or because the uterus hasn't contracted after the placenta has been delivered. Even in a country with good medical care, a postpartum haemorrhage is a frightening experience.

Labours that have resulted in the baby dying or being severely disabled often lead to birth trauma. This was the case for Miriam. Her third baby was delivered at 31 weeks of pregnancy when she suffered an abrupted placenta, which means that the placenta separated from her uterus and caused her to haemorrhage. The baby had to be delivered quickly by caesarean section. Miriam was taken to theatre and given an epidural. However, they started operating on her before the epidural took effect, and so then had to deliver the baby under general anaesthetic.

Miriam had to be given two blood transfusions, after which she stopped breathing, and had to be put on life support, but she recovered. Her baby, Ruth, seemed healthy at first, but later developed chronic lung disease, and Miriam and her husband went through the traumatic experience of finding that the baby had stopped breathing and having to carry out CPR on her before she was taken back to hospital. As her parents were coming to terms with having to manage a chronic lung condition, Ruth was diagnosed with Down's Syndrome. For the first year of Ruth's life, Miriam said she was stressed and anxious, but it was only when her lung condition started to get slightly better that the full force of the diagnosis and everything she'd been through finally hit her and she 'crashed':

'I was waking up in the night with panic attacks and had to calm myself down in the morning, felt on red alert all the time and the only things that would turn things down a notch were Diazepam or wine, so I drank too much wine in the evenings, and felt very anxious if I was separated from Ruth or the other children. I had flashbacks as well to the delivery time and to the time of Ruth's diagnosis and the time she stopped breathing. I think what hit me was the full horror of what happened when at the time I just had to get on with it.'

Although the fear of dying, or fear that the baby will die, are the key components in birth trauma, there are other factors that can add to the trauma, or make it more likely that you will experience trauma symptoms.

Research suggests that women who suffer birth trauma have often had long, difficult labours (or sometimes, very short, intense ones), or a highly medicalised delivery, involving forceps or emergency caesarean. Many women report feeling a loss of control, or having their pain dismissed by unsympathetic medical staff.

Professor Cheryl Beck, an academic who has carried out research into birth trauma, writes:

> 'A high level of obstetric intervention during childbirth and the perception of inadequate labor and delivery care were associated significantly with the development of acute trauma symptoms.'[5]

Similarly, one study of six couples who had suffered birth trauma found that every participant commented on poor quality of care during birth, typically a lack of information, staff incompetence or indifference, or a lack of continuity of care.[6]

Jane Canning is a midwife who works for Birth Stories, a service offered by Brighton and Sussex University Hospitals Trust that enables women to talk through their difficult birth experiences. She says there are some common features in the women who use their service:

> 'We see a lot of women having their first babies with slow progress, leading to prolonged and often, painful labour and lots of interventions. Long labours and quick labours may both be experienced as traumatic. I think women can feel there is a lack of participation in decision-making. During a long labour, when interventions become necessary, suddenly lots is happening for them, especially when delivery is needed promptly and women commonly refer to feeling invisible, unseen or unheard.'

Violeta, whose two-day labour was followed by an emergency caesarean and a postpartum haemorrhage, says:

> 'Most of the staff treated me with kindness and professionalism. One midwife did not – she hurt me during an internal examination, broke my waters without telling me, failed to act with kindness and a minimum of sympathy,

failed to offer pain relief and was dismissive. Her behaviour and words are the cause of much of my PTSD.'

Sally had both a midwife and a trainee present at her birth. She felt the midwife didn't listen to her or explain what was happening:

'I had internal monitoring and they started to get concerned about his heart rate. I remember the midwife telling me she didn't have time to explain but they were very concerned about my baby and to do what she said. They told me to move position but didn't help me and I had nothing to brace myself on…The pain was very bad and unpredictable and although I kept telling them they weren't regular, sometimes the midwife took the gas and air away as a contraction was coming because she thought it wasn't one. This added to my feelings that I couldn't trust her. She also kept saying, "I know what you want, I've read your birth plan. I know you want X and don't want Y" about things that weren't in my birth plan, which made me wonder if she was confusing me with someone or was just useless.'

Sally was then told the baby had to be delivered quickly because its life was at risk:

'The midwife wanted to do an episiotomy and, although I had read papers suggesting it was better to tear for various reasons, I agreed – anything to get him out as I felt his life was in danger. The pain was so bad I felt I would do anything to get it to end. But I was also very scared my baby was dead and no-one was telling me what was going on.'

Despite this apparent worry about the baby's safety, Sally's baby was delivered by the trainee:

'I never consented to this. And if they were so concerned about his heart rate why would you let an inexperienced trainee deliver him?'

Charise, who suffered a haemorrhage requiring four blood transfusions after an already difficult labour, felt that she was kept in the dark for much of the time:

'When the pain got too much I told them I was ready to go upstairs [to the delivery ward]. They said "No, we will put you on a monitor and see how you're getting on in an hour." I was in agony in my side, I lay on the bed and when I lay on one side my baby's heart rate was dropping dangerously low. Then they put me on the other side and it came back up again, again with no explanation of why. They just told me not to lie on that side.'

Frequently women with birth trauma describe having their complaints or questions ignored during labour. Charise had been sure there was something wrong during her labour:

'They weren't listening. I was telling them for hours, "There's something wrong, there's something wrong," and I knew there was something wrong, something didn't feel right. It was the third time I've given birth and it wasn't the same. But you can't say "I've got a pain here", because they're like, "You'll have a pain everywhere, darling, you're in labour." I kept mentioning it over and over again, but they weren't listening to me.'

For some women the physical demands and extreme pain of labour can lead to trauma symptoms, particularly if they are not adequately supported by staff. Several women I spoke to for this book had been denied pain relief or other interventions when they desperately needed them.

Nina's labour lasted for 42 hours and was marked by a series of stressful events – at one point, staff couldn't find a heartbeat and thought the baby had died. During much of her labour, she found the pain agonising and asked for an epidural, but wasn't given one until two hours before the baby was born. A midwife had tried to carry out an internal examination, but had failed because Nina had a tilted cervix (a fairly common condition in which the uterus is tipped back rather than forwards). She thinks this is perhaps why the epidural was refused, though this wasn't explained to her. At one point she was given the painkiller pethidine, which made her fall asleep, but her memory of what happened during the hours of pain that followed is unclear. Her husband, Jon, talked to her afterwards about what had happened:

'I instantly woke up screaming, because the thing about pethidine is, it doesn't stop the pain. What happened for the rest of the night was that Jon said I was like a really naughty drunk person, who would be trying to push the buttons on the machines and get out of bed, and wander off, but then every time I had a contraction, I'd be screaming and go over to the window so I could throw myself out. It's a blessing that I can't remember much of it.'

Jon told Nina that he had asked for her to be given further pain relief:

'I asked him: "Did you say at any point, Look at the state she's in, can you give her anything?" and he said, "I asked, but they said there's nothing they could do." And he's not a passive person. He's very much an advocate for me. He was very distressed and not coping very well, but if there was anything he could have made them do he'd have made them do it.

'I was delirious because of the pain, and I didn't know you could be delirious through pain, I didn't know that could happen. And I kept having the recurring thought which was, "When people are in car crashes, they pass out, so why am I still conscious?" I guess it's biology, your body needs you to be conscious. But that was the one thought I kept having.'

Women who suffer from birth trauma often describe feeling out of control and not knowing what is happening to them. In Nina's words:

'I was out of control because the pain and pethidine sent you crazy.'

Risk factors
Some women are more predisposed to experience birth trauma if they've had a traumatic experience in the past, such as rape or sexual abuse, for example. One research paper says:

'The labour itself could awaken feelings and triggers associated with the original trauma, possibly because the woman will feel vulnerable, out of control and experience pain.'[7]

Sometimes they have a specific fear relating to giving birth. In Rebecca's case, it was a fear of needles:

'I felt increasingly anxious during the pregnancy and couldn't actually imagine giving birth in a hospital, as I knew I would feel massively anxious about any medical procedures, I used to make myself feel ill imagining episiotomies.'

Rebecca was in labour for two days before she reached the pushing stage:

'Into my third day of labour, I pushed for over two hours before it was decided I was too exhausted to birth naturally. They shouted at me to agree to an episiotomy and Ventouse – which was correct, I did need one but was so terrified I wouldn't agree – and so one was performed, an injection then cut, and she was pulled out. The pain was appalling, as was the butcher's shop of the room left behind afterwards. Being sewn up in the vaginal area was deeply traumatic to me – not sure much anaesthetic was used – due to this being my worst fear of all time, although the stitches did heal well afterwards. In my head, I was being attacked in a very visceral way.'

Afterwards she experienced flashbacks to 'the worst part of the birth, in which I felt my baby being dragged out, and the sewing.' Very often, however, women who experience birth trauma have no history to suggest they are predisposed to suffer from it.

Is birth trauma different from other forms of PTSD?
Although the same criteria are used for diagnosing birth trauma as for PTSD after other traumatic events, Dr Antje Horsch, a clinical psychologist who has researched birth trauma, argues that it has three particular features that make it distinctive:

♦ In most causes of PTSD (such as a car accident, or a violent attack), the event is unexpected. In birth trauma, however, the event is something that women have usually looked forward to. At some point while the woman is giving birth, her view of the event changes from being positive to being negative. 'Usually with a traumatic event, it just happens out of the blue, completely unexpectedly,' says Dr Horsch. 'In contrast childbirth is something women anticipate for a long time and anticipate with lots of joy and positive feelings, so at some point there is some transformation that takes place from a positive to a negative event.'

19

♦ In a traumatic birth, there are two people involved, the mother and the baby. Usually (though not always), PTSD sufferers are able to avoid some of the reminders of the traumatic event. When a woman has given birth, however, she has to live with the baby, who will be a constant reminder of the traumatic birth. 'Immediately after the baby is born, the mother is forced to forge a close relationship to this baby, and the baby is completely dependent on the mother, so that's also very different from other types of trauma,' says Dr Horsch.

♦ Normally PTSD sufferers are not expected to go through the traumatic event again. If you're in a car crash, nobody expects you to undergo another car crash. Yet many women, having had a traumatic birth, will want to have another baby, says Dr Horsch: 'Ultimately women are forced back to go through this again, so in some ways it's inevitable if they want to have more children, they have to face this again.'

How many women suffer from birth trauma?
Estimates of the prevalence of birth trauma range from 1.5% to 6% of women who give birth. These are rough estimates – it is hard to know exactly how many women suffer from PTSD, as not all seek help.

About 700,000 women give birth each year in England and Wales. At the low end (1.5%), this translates into about 10,000 women a year going on to experience full-blown PTSD – that is, they match all the diagnostic criteria. Many more experience some PTSD symptoms. One survey of mothers in the United States found that 9% of them appeared to meet all the formal criteria for post-traumatic stress disorder, much higher than we might expect.[8] A more recent Israeli survey of 89 women found that three suffered full-blown PTSD, while a quarter had some symptoms but were not considered to have PTSD.[9]

Because birth trauma has only been recognised as a condition in very recent years (and even now, not everyone is convinced of its existence), it's difficult to say whether the incidence is increasing. There is a case for arguing that the process of birth is becoming more difficult for women in developed countries, as a result of certain trends: babies are getting bigger, women are giving birth at an older age, more women are having IVF, and more women are obese, often with related conditions such as diabetes or heart problems. All these can make birth more risky. However, there is no conclusive evidence to show that these trends have increased the incidence of birth trauma.

As awareness of the condition increases, it seems likely that more women will receive a formal diagnosis. Even now, many women who do not meet the full diagnostic criteria do still suffer PTSD symptoms after giving birth and could benefit from professional help.

What are the symptoms of birth trauma?

The symptoms of birth trauma are the same as for PTSD following any traumatic event. The four characteristic symptoms are re-experiencing the trauma, avoidance, negative cognitions and mood, and arousal.

Re-experiencing the trauma: flashbacks, nightmares and intrusive memories
People who have been through a traumatic experience find themselves reliving it over and over again. 'At the heart of PTSD lie involuntary re-living experiences (intrusive thoughts, nightmares, flashbacks)' writes Dr Antje Horsch.[10]

Intrusive memories are memories of the event that appear unbidden in the mind. Flashbacks are similar to intrusive memories, but they make the sufferer feel as if the event is happening all over again, and may even be accompanied by smells or sounds.

During a flashback, sufferers may feel the same emotions and sense of panic that they experienced at the time. These feelings can be intensely distressing, and are sometimes accompanied by physical reactions, such as a pounding heart or sweating.

Some people have nightmares either of the event or other frightening scenarios:

'I am prone to dark thoughts, which started after my daughter was born. They are related to the flashbacks – when I was flashbacking I could really feel it, and then it moved onto dreams of my daughter being taken away or hurt badly or killed.' (Sarah)

Michelle started to lose blood after giving birth, but the midwife seemed unconcerned. Lying on the floor, she was told by the midwife to get on the bed. She tried, and fainted, and then began to haemorrhage more badly, eventually losing four pints of blood. Later, scenes from the birth and the immediate aftermath would play out over and over again in her mind:

'I kept on having these visions of me lying on the floor and looking at David with him holding Ivy. There are three images from that scene: me collapsing back after saying, "I can't get up", and them saying "You should"; and then looking around after coming round and seeing him; and then afterwards on the bed, looking at Ivy and thinking, "Oh my God, I've got to look after her now, and I don't even want her." I'm posing for pictures, and trying to smile and look happy and thinking, "I can't be bothered".'

One woman, Evie, had a highly atypical experience, in that she didn't realise she was pregnant until she started to give birth. For her the trauma was connected to the shock of discovering she was having a baby:

'I couldn't shake my nightmares. Constantly thinking about what could have happened, and remembering the absolute terror that I felt when I looked down and saw a tiny hand.'

There is a clear contrast between the way memory is processed in women who experience PTSD after birth and those who don't. In a study by Susan Ayers of women who had been through traumatic births, the women who didn't go on to develop PTSD symptoms often described forgetting how bad the experience was.[11] One said:

'I forget everything about it, you know, I don't remember anything.'

For those women who did develop PTSD symptoms, parts (though not all) of the birth experience remained very vivid in the memory.

Avoidance

People who have PTSD may go out of their way to avoid anything that reminds them of the traumatic event. Emma, for example, avoided situations where she might hear people talk about birth, and couldn't bring herself to watch programmes about birth. Often women who have had a traumatic birth avoid returning to the hospital where they gave birth, even for check-ups:

'Any time I watched anything to do with birth, any time anyone mentioned anything to do with birth or babies, I'd start shaking and get really weepy and upset. When I went to have a scan, a normal 12-week scan with my second child four years later, I was having a panic attack, in the waiting room and I had a panic attack on the way out again, because I couldn't deal with the fact that I was going back into a hospital, though it was a different hospital. I steered clear of doctors and hospitals for about four years.' (Sarah)

'There was a lot of guilt about it, and anger. I couldn't really let it go. I talked about it all the time, but also found it very difficult to listen to other people's stories.' (Alice)

Sometimes this avoidance is accompanied by a general lack of interest in life and an emotional numbness. Some women find they cannot develop an emotional attachment to their baby. After a very difficult birth, Sally says:

'I didn't bond at all with my son. He just felt like an alien I had to look after.'

Dr Ayers says that avoidance tends to be slightly less common among mothers than among other PTSD sufferers, perhaps because the presence of the baby is a constant reminder of the experience of giving birth.

Negative cognitions and mood

This is a new diagnostic criterion for PTSD, included for the first time in DSM-5. It covers a wide spectrum of feelings, including 'a persistent and distorted sense of blame of self or others, to estrangement from others or markedly diminished interest in activities to an inability to remember key aspects of the event.'[12] Nina, for example, has no recollection of trying to throw herself out of the window and had to rely on her husband to fill in the gaps. Charise found herself becoming very withdrawn:

'I suffer with insomnia anyway in times of stress, and I couldn't sleep at all. I was getting maybe two or three hours during the day, and in the night I wasn't getting any sleep at all. I had really bad panic attacks. I didn't like going out without my husband, I didn't want to see any-body. I didn't want any visitors or anything. I just became very insular and I just wasn't myself really.'

Arousal

PTSD sufferers often experience increased emotional arousal: they are more anxious and more alert. They may feel irritable or find it difficult to concentrate or to fall asleep. Sometimes this arousal takes the form of hyper-vigilance, which is an increased anxiety or fearfulness. Someone who has been the victim of a violent crime, for example, may always be looking around for escape routes. In cases of PTSD after giving birth, this usually manifests itself in a greater anxiety about the baby. Nina, who suffered from birth trauma after a long, painful and often frightening labour, became particularly anxious once she was home:

> 'My adrenaline was constantly going, I was constantly angry or constantly on the verge of a panic attack, or constantly being vigilant in case baby wanted anything, and I was like that for so long it became normal.'

The anxiety extended to keeping the baby clean:

> 'I got very strange about her cleanliness. If some things were dirty or contaminated they had to be thrown away, not touched. I was very worried about the contamination of the baby. I didn't like people touching her.'

Other symptoms

Although re-experiencing the event, avoidance, negative cognitions and mood, and arousal are the four symptoms that will lead to a diagnosis of PTSD, many sufferers report feeling guilty and think it must be their fault that the birth has gone wrong:

> 'I loved her from the very moment she was born, but I felt I'd let her down so badly because I wasn't able to look after her.' (Emma)

'I had a lot of guilt, and I felt like a terrible mother, and a terrible wife and like a failure because women are meant to have babies and women have much worse things than this happen to them. They have babies who die and all sorts and they don't get PTSD so I felt really weak.' (Nina)

'I had no problems with bonding with the baby, but the guilt was there, a lot of guilt that I hadn't done enough to make sure he was OK.' (Alice)

The guilt can be particularly strong if the woman had been planning a normal delivery:

'I didn't want to talk to the doctor about it. I felt really ashamed that I hadn't managed to have a natural birth.' (Sarah)

Some PTSD sufferers also experience dissociation – a feeling that you have lost touch with what is happening around you, or that you are outside your own body.

How long do symptoms last?

PTSD symptoms can start quite soon after the birth. In some women, the symptoms will disappear spontaneously. Although there hasn't been research into how long PTSD symptoms typically last with women who experience them after giving birth, research into rape victims shows that about 96% experience PTSD symptoms immediately after the rape, but the figure drops to half that after three months.[13]

Maureen Treadwell, co-founder of the Birth Trauma Association (BTA), says that when the organisation was first launched in 2004, it was approached by women in their 50s who still hadn't recovered from trauma that had been untreated 20 or 30 years previously. One woman writing on the Mumsnet internet forum said that she still experienced flashbacks 42 years after her son was born.

Triggers

There are certain situations that can trigger PTSD symptoms again, even if the woman otherwise seems to have recovered from them. Sexual intimacy can be one of the triggers, but there are others. Alice found certain things always reminded her of the birth:

'Sometimes if I leant over the cot, standing up, it reminded me of being leant over while I was in labour. I had a dressing gown, and that hadn't been worn so I'd brought it home, but then I couldn't look at it, I had to throw it away.'

Some women fear visiting the hospital where they gave birth because they know it will distress them. In her second pregnancy, Alice had to return to the same hospital where she'd had a bad experience first time around:

'I had to go to the hospital for a gynae appointment not long ago, and it's in the same part of the hospital. Even then it would take me straight back to being on that corridor. When I was going to have my second child, I point blank refused. I said I would not go onto that antenatal ward. I can't go there, I just wouldn't go there.'

For Rebecca, becoming pregnant a second time a year after the birth of her first child acted as a trigger. The flashbacks intensified:

'I used to lie there, trying to sleep, thinking about the awfulness of the last birth and about all the likely (in my fevered imagination) things that would happen in the second. It was like watching myself in a horror film with myself in the starring role.'

Internal examinations and smear tests can also be strong triggers. Nina, who was called for a smear test when her baby was three years old, found the experience distressing:

'Prior to the appointment I didn't want to think about anything PTSD-related as I was trying to put it out of my mind, and after the appointment I was in a bit of a state and felt sad and upset for a week or so – I suppose it just raked up old feelings that would have been better left alone. Thank heavens the nurse who did the test was very kind and understanding. She even apologised for what happened to me previously on behalf of nurses and gave me a big hug at the end – it didn't stop me from wailing like a banshee throughout and shaking so much I almost fell off the trolley, though.'

Postnatal depression and PTSD

Birth trauma is often accompanied by postnatal depression (PND). More than 50% of women who suffer birth trauma also get symptoms of depression. Sarah experienced both – though she did not seek professional help:

'When I did the Edinburgh postnatal survey, one of the questions was about suicidal thoughts, and at that point I thought, "What I've been having is not normal", because I remember lying in the bath and looking at the razors, and thinking, 'How can I take this apart?" and I could feel it in my skin, what it would feel like. We lived by the sea, so I'd taken my daughter up to the top of the cliff and had a really black day, and I thought, "I could throw myself over now and nobody would miss me".'

Health professionals are usually much better, however, at identifying PND than they are at identifying birth trauma. Health visitors now routinely administer the Edinburgh Postnatal Depression Scale to women a few weeks after birth. This will pick up cases of PND (if women answer it honestly) but not birth trauma. Although a PTSD diagnostic scale exists for diagnosing PTSD, it is not routinely administered in the same way as the Edinburgh scale. Unfortunately, there is still a lot of ignorance, even among health professionals, about PTSD after birth, so some GPs will misdiagnose birth trauma as depression:

> 'Midwives told me not to think about it and just get on with life. A trainee GP was very helpful and sympathetic when my husband tried to get some help but she didn't know where to go for help. The health visitor was very patronising. Everyone seemed to think it was PND.' (Sally)

> 'I cried every day for the first month after she was born, and was assessed by a mental health team about two weeks after birth, although they were not massively concerned beyond that I was a candidate for PND and was offered antidepressants which I did not take.' (Rebecca)

Misdiagnosis can be problematic, because the most common treatment for depression is anti-depressants, usually SSRIs, and while these can be effective in treating PND, they are not usually helpful in treating birth trauma, and may even make it worse. The National Institute for Health and Care Excellence (NICE) researches evidence into treatments, and publishes guidelines for doctors about how to treat particular illnesses. The guidelines it has produced on treating PTSD recommend the use of trauma-focused psychological therapies to treat the condition. They say:

> 'Drug treatments for PTSD should not be used as a routine first-line treatment for adults (in general use or by

specialist mental health professionals) in preference to a trauma-focused psychological therapy.'[14]

The situation is more complicated if a patient has both PTSD and PND. A good therapist will be able to treat both. The NICE guidelines acknowledge, however, that when the sufferer has both PTSD and depression there may be a case for offering certain kinds of antidepressant to treat the depression.

Chapter 4 gives more information about the treatments available for birth trauma.

Is birth trauma avoidable?

This is not an easy question to answer. Some women are at risk of experiencing birth trauma because they have experienced a previous trauma. One way of reducing the incidence of birth trauma might be to identify at-risk women beforehand and to offer them the support they need. Midwives would have to be trained to do this effectively. Some women may feel unhappy answering questions about previous traumatic experiences, particularly if these questions are not asked in a sensitive manner.

Many women, however, are not obviously at risk. We do not know yet why some women who have a difficult birth don't go on to develop birth trauma, while others do. Some people believe that if a woman has planned a normal birth, the mismatch between what she'd imagined and the reality of a difficult labour with medical interventions may be especially traumatic. However, this doesn't seem to be borne out by the evidence.[15]

A common theme among many women who turn to the BTA for support, says Maureen Treadwell, is that they've felt a 'lack of control' during labour: staff haven't explained to them what is happening, or not responded to their requests for pain relief. 'There is no other area of healthcare where people are routinely left in that level of pain,' Maureen points out. Part of the work that the BTA does is to educate health professionals to listen to what women want and to take their views into account, rather than assuming that a birth without pain relief is necessarily the best outcome. Elizabeth Ford, a psychology researcher, writes that:

'It may not be the level of pain per se which is traumatising for women, but the experience of unbearable pain in combination with the perception of being denied pain-relief by an uncooperative caregiver.'[16]

As we saw earlier, the other issue that frequently crops up in research studies is that women feel they have been kept in the dark about what is happening to them, and the resulting confusion and fear play a part in the subsequent birth trauma. Health professionals could address this by taking a more patient-centred approach. Jean Robinson, president of the Alliance for Improvement in Maternity Services (AIMS), argues persuasively that obstetricians and midwives should receive training on women's psychological vulnerability when they are giving birth.[17]

We should also, perhaps, recognise that even when it goes well, giving birth is an intensely physical and emotional experience, and quite unlike anything else that most of us will experience during our lives. As Jane Canning says:

'Birth is such a powerful experience, and the impact on women is huge. I think that women can be left with many questions and unresolved feelings relating to this experience.'

***

Louise's story

Louise gave birth in Spain, where she was living with her husband. She knew she was going to have a big baby: two weeks before she gave birth, her waistline was 50 inches and she asked staff for a caesarean, which was refused. The baby was two weeks overdue and Louise was induced with prostaglandin pessaries. After 24 hours of first-stage back-to-back labour (where the baby is facing forwards instead of backwards, making labour more painful), she wasn't progressing, so Louise was given Syntocinon, a synthetic hormone that made the contractions more frequent and intense. Louise was also given pethidine for pain relief but found it didn't help:

'I was so stoned on it, I couldn't even articulate how much in pain I was. I found that really stressful. I was just talking a load of nonsense, I really didn't like it.'

Although Louise repeatedly asked for a caesarean section, she wasn't allowed one:

'I felt nobody would help me,' she says. 'I felt completely defenceless. It could have taken another 10 hours and they just didn't care enough. It was just obscene because there is a ward on the floor below and the floor above, and they won't help you, they won't take you there, and sort it out, they make you go through it like an animal in the field.'

Six hours later, Louise was given an epidural, and three hours after that she began pushing the baby out – a process that took another four hours, and at the end of which she gave birth to an 11lb baby boy. The entire labour had lasted 37 hours.

After the birth, Louise lost a lot of blood, but wasn't given a transfusion. The effort of pushing the baby out led to her damaging a nerve in her neck, which gave her intense headaches for a month afterwards.

'They were so bad that I had to wear glasses all the time, even if it was dark,' she says. She also had painful episiotomy stitches: 'I was a complete physical wreck. I couldn't walk, I couldn't breastfeed, I couldn't take my glasses off.'

She started to develop symptoms of PTSD:

'I put on something like five stone when I was pregnant. I lost it really quickly, because I was so stressed. I was having night sweats, I couldn't sleep, I was smoking like a chimney, not in front of the baby, but I went into a real manic episode for about six months.'

Louise also found it difficult to develop a bond with her baby:

'The first few weeks home I could hardly bear to look at him, I was so traumatised.'

In Spain, there are no home visits from midwives after birth. Although she was prescribed antidepressants by her doctor, Louise was not offered counselling, and feels that health professionals were to a large extent unconcerned:

'No one gave a damn about my mental health – all I got was, "You've got a damaged nerve in your neck" and "You should be breastfeeding."'

At the same time, Louise felt angry with her husband for not fighting her corner more at the hospital and pushing for a caesarean, though she also recognises that this was hard for him to do, as in Spain, heath professionals 'are very quick to whisk difficult fathers off the ward entirely.'

An important turning-point came at six months, when the baby was baptised:

'When we had baptised him, which was culturally important for us, it was actually quite healing. After that I stopped having the night sweats.'

Recovery from birth trauma has been gradual – it has taken nearly two years for Louise to feel able to talk about her experience openly. During that time she has also been able to develop a closer bond with her baby:

'I'm always trying to make up for the fact that for the first few months of his life I wasn't particularly loving, I didn't get any joy from having a baby which is the sad thing. People talk about having a big rush of love. I didn't feel that, I just felt relief.'

Louise managed to overcome her trauma enough to decide to have a second baby. She had a far happier experience second time round. Back in the UK, Louise received regular counseling sessions from the NHS while pregnant, which helped her feel calmer and more confident. She regards the second birth, by planned caesarean section, as 'the best day of my life', adding, 'the single thing I have done to recover from the first birth has been giving birth to my second, and I feel as though a great sadness has lifted from me'.

Chapter 2: You and your baby

If you have been through a traumatic birth, it is probably not surprising that you feel indifferent or resentful, or even actively hostile, towards your baby. It is the baby, after all, who has been the cause of your suffering, and 'avoidance' – staying away from anything that reminds you of the trauma – is a key component of PTSD.

In one study of mothers with PTSD, several women reported that their early feelings towards their baby were hostile.[1] One said:

> 'I can remember thinking, you horrible thing, you've done this to me, and what are you doing here, you evil child.'

Another reported thinking:

> 'In God's name why are you giving me a baby, you know, I'm dying, why would I want a baby?'

She even felt the baby rejected her:

> 'The baby had one eye open, one closed, and he looked at me and there was this scowl on his face as if to say, where am I and in God's name don't tell me you're my mother.'

This is a far cry from what women expect to feel when their baby is born. Many women expect to 'bond' instantly with their baby, and if this doesn't happen, then the guilt about not bonding can add to the misery of the birth trauma, which in turn makes them feel even more distant from the baby. Without support, it's easy to become trapped in a vicious circle.

Most women do eventually bond with their baby – but for some it takes longer than others. This chapter looks at what bonding is, why it matters, and whether there are techniques that can help you bond.

Attachment and bonding

The term attachment was first used by the psychologist John Bowlby, who believed that babies are born with a biological need to become 'attached' to one person, and that mothers have a similar need to stay in close contact with their baby.[2] This instinctive connection between mother and baby has evolved to improve the baby's chances of survival. A baby's behaviour stimulates an appropriate response in the mother – if the baby cries, for example, the mother will pick it up and cuddle it or feed it.

Dr Bruce Perry, an expert on child mental health, explains attachment like this:

> 'An emotionally and physically healthy mother will be drawn to her infant — she will feel a physical longing to smell, cuddle, rock, coo, and gaze at her infant. In turn the infant will respond with snuggling, babbling, smiling, sucking, and clinging. In most cases, the mother's behaviors bring pleasure and nourishment to the infant, and the infant's behaviors bring pleasure and satisfaction to the mother. This reciprocal positive feedback loop, this maternal-infant dance, is where attachment develops.'[3]

Psychologists use the term 'bonding' to describe the process by which the baby and mother form an attachment.

Not all mothers bond instantly with their baby, however. Even some mothers who haven't suffered birth trauma or PND sometimes find it hard to bond, though we don't know exact numbers. According to psychologist Sarah Helps:

> 'Bonding and attachment are pretty much automatic processes, but there are times when it goes awry, when it

doesn't go quite as smoothly. Things like postnatal depression can get in the way, things like external stress, issues to do with the baby, issues to do with what's going on for the mum or issues to do with what's going on around the mum can all serve to complicate the bonding and attachment process.'[4]

How birth trauma can make it hard to bond
Bonding with a new baby can be difficult when you are suffering from birth trauma. Your feelings towards the baby may be inseparable from the terrible experience you had of giving birth, and you may want to avoid reminders of the birth. If the baby has been hurt during the birth, or is ill or disabled, or has been kept separately from you during the hours, days or even weeks following birth, this can exacerbate feelings of loss or guilt or anger, or simply a sense of remoteness from the baby. PND, which often accompanies birth trauma, can also hinder bonding.

Some people think that the normal bonding process can be disrupted by a lack of the hormone oxytocin. As well as helping the uterus contract in labour, oxytocin, sometimes jokingly referred to as the 'love' hormone, seems to play a role in making the mother feel calm and relaxed and helping her bond with her baby. During a traumatic labour, the body releases the stress hormones adrenaline and cortisol, and it may be that these reduce the flow of oxytocin, so that instead of feeling warm and relaxed, the new mother still feels stressed and anxious.

Psychologist Susan Ayers, who has carried out research into how women with birth trauma bond with their babies, says her studies showed two different patterns:

'Some women rejected the baby, which is what you'd expect with the avoidance symptoms. If the woman associates the baby with the birth, it makes sense that she will try and avoid the baby because she will want to avoid any reminders of the birth, that's how the logic goes... But then other women almost went the other way and became over-anxiously protective of the baby.'

Evie, who hadn't known she was pregnant until she was in second stage labour, initially felt nothing for her daughter when she was born:

'I was unsure whether I wanted to keep her. I didn't want her anywhere near me. I was in total shock and couldn't tell anyone even my name for two days.'

For about 11 months, Evie suffered from postnatal depression (PND) as well as trauma symptoms: 'I found I didn't love her the way I should and was just caring for her because I felt I had to.'

The ability to have early skin-to-skin contact with the baby is an important part of the bonding process, and if the birth has been difficult, this often doesn't happen. Charise, who had short-term problems bonding with her baby, had to be rushed to the operating theatre for a blood transfusion when her son was born:

'I felt like I'd missed out on being the first. I didn't get him dressed – I was wheeled away to theatre, and my husband was handed a naked baby, and when I came back he was dressed and wrapped in a blanket and asleep in a bed, which I was really upset about. I didn't get to feed him first because he was in special care, and they fed him, so I was upset about that.'

Initially her baby had health problems, which he later recovered from:

'He's perfect now, there's nothing wrong with him at all, he's absolutely fine. I'm very protective of him and I don't like him going to other people's houses and things, I don't like to be away from him for very long.'

While some women find it difficult to bond with their baby, others, as Dr Ayers points out, go to the opposite extreme – they become anxious and over-protective. This anxiety is a feature of the 'hyper-vigilance' that often characterises PTSD. For Nina, anxiety about the baby was mixed up with feelings of rage and despair:

'When Jon went back to work, I was very angry that he had a life and I didn't have a life, and I just felt, although I loved her so much, "What have I done? I've ruined my life. Absolutely ruined my life". And then there was a song on the radio at the time that went "I want my life back, I want my life back". Left alone in the house with a baby, I would think, "What do I do with her?" I bought swinging chairs and things for the baby, but I'd put her in it and because she was a baby, she wasn't familiar with it, she'd cry and I wouldn't put her in it again because I was almost phobic about her crying, I would avoid anything that would upset her. For me a good day was a day she hadn't cried, and I literally had days where she didn't cry. Because I watched her, and as soon as she wanted anything, I did it. She didn't have chance to cry.'

Nina's experience was similar to that of a woman quoted in a study by Karen Nicholls and Susan Ayers:

'I think it's made me so overprotective of her. I don't let her out of my sight. I don't like other people touching her... I mean my mum...obviously I trust her with her, but I'd go out to the pub with my sister and after half an hour later I'd have to go home again because I was so frightened about what would happen to [the baby]... I had to go back. I just can't bear it, it's just really frightening.'[5]

Birth trauma is complicated, so it's not always the case that you feel either indifferent or over-protective towards your baby. Some women feel both. Sally had a bad labour during which she had lost trust in the midwives. Like many women she felt exhilarated once the baby was born:

> 'I felt on quite a high, relieved it was over and he was okay. Instead of this adrenaline feeling fading I felt more and more charged up as time went on. I had an overwhelming urge to pick up my baby and run and run and run. This carried on for a long time.'

Once she was at home with the baby, she hoped life would get back to normal, but it didn't:

> 'I blocked out everything to do with the labour and just wanted to get on with things. But I felt so anxious, I couldn't leave him on his own. I had a huge feeling of dread, premonitions that something bad was going to happen to him. I knew it was going to happen but didn't know how it was going to happen so I was on the lookout for any source of danger, including myself. I couldn't sleep at all for a long time.'

At the same time as feeling this anxiety, she began to lose the connection she'd initially felt with her son:

> 'I felt something for him when he was born but it seemed to disappear. I asked my husband how he felt about him and he said his feelings were growing, while I felt I'd lost anything positive I felt about him.'

For a new mother, the experience of feeling nothing for one's new baby can be hugely distressing. Professor Cheryl Beck quotes one mother who suffered birth trauma after an unplanned caesarean section:

'At night I tried to connect/acknowledge in my heart that this was my son and I cried. I knew that there were great layers of trauma around my heart. I wanted to feel motherhood. I wanted to experience and embrace it.'[6]

This woman's sense of loss was overwhelming – she describes herself as feeling 'chained up in the viselike grip of this pain.'

How long does it take to bond?

If you do have difficulties bonding with your baby as a result of birth trauma, these normally fade with time. Dr Helen Barrett, a research psychologist, points out that many mothers (not just those with birth trauma) develop a closer relationship with their children once they have passed the baby stage.

It does seem to vary, however. In one study of mothers with birth trauma, Cheryl Beck looked at how the baby's first birthday can serve to reawaken disturbing memories of the birth and even reinforce mothers' feelings of distance from their child.[7] One woman said:

'As my daughter's first birthday approached I wanted to die. I felt nothing for her and found it hard to celebrate the joy of this child that meant so little to me. I took excellent care of her but it was if I was babysitting, the emotional bond just wasn't there.'

For another, the feelings continued well past the first birthday:

'Each year as my daughter's birthday approaches I feel more and more anxious. I have a strong belief that her real parents will turn up and demand to know why I had been so bad at looking after their child.'

Some women (though by no means all) felt much relaxed at the second or subsequent birthday, and one woman in Beck's study described her daughter's second birthday party as the 'most joyful time I've ever had'. In the Nicholls and Ayers study, most of the women felt rejection towards their baby at the beginning but bonded over a period of one to five years.[8]

This was also true for the women who spoke to me for this book – all of them eventually grew to love and care for their babies:

> 'It took me about six months to feel "love" for my baby. I felt huge responsibility towards him from the beginning, but didn't fall in love immediately.' (Violeta)

Evie, shocked and traumatised by an unexpected birth, eventually grew to love her baby and is glad she made the decision to keep her.

It's likely, however, that a minority of women never succeed in bonding with their children, which is why it's hugely important that women experiencing birth trauma are offered help as early as possible.

Will it harm my baby if I don't bond immediately?

It would be good to be able to give a straightforward 'yes' or 'no' answer to this question. In fact, the real picture is complicated, not least because research into birth trauma is relatively new, so there haven't been any long-term studies into the impact of a mother's birth trauma on her baby's development.

Some psychologists argue that early bonding is crucial, and that babies' brain development is permanently shaped by their early experiences. Sue Gerhardt's book *Why love matters* cites recent research on neuroscience to support the view that how a mother behaves towards her baby in the early months has a lifelong impact on that baby's development.[9] Raised levels of the stress hormone cortisol, for example, have been found in babies left alone for long periods, and high levels of cortisol are associated with depression and anxiety. Gerhardt describes the importance of attachment in strong terms:

> 'Babies need a caregiver who identifies with them so strongly that the baby's needs feel like hers; he is still physiologically and psychologically an extension of her. If she feels bad when the baby feels bad, she will then want to do something about it immediately, to relieve the baby's discomfort.'

Conversely, she argues, a mother who doesn't respond instinctively in this way risks raising a child who is unhappy and anxious in later life. One long-term study found that children of women who suffer from PND are more than three times as likely as other children to suffer from depression by the time they are 16, and that this is linked to poor attachment in infancy.[10]

The thought that, if you don't form a close attachment with your baby in the early weeks, he may grow up to be an unhappy or depressed adult, is a scary one for any mother who hasn't felt that rush of love for her baby. But not all psychologists are convinced. In her book *Attachment and the perils of parenting*, Dr Barrett makes a different case, arguing that there is a lack of good evidence to support Gerhardt's views:[11]

> 'The small number of longitudinal studies of attachment behaviour across the lifespan do not support the notion that attachment patterns are fixed and unchangeable from early on...Many assertions about what neuroscience is showing are over-simplifications...We still don't know enough to be sure of what the links are between early experience, brain development and patterns of attachment.'

In other words, even if you don't form a close bond with your baby in the first few months, this doesn't necessarily affect your child adversely in the long term – there may be time to bond as your baby grows older. Dr Barrett points out that even John Bowlby, the father of attachment theory, revised his earlier views to suggest that children could still form strong attachments after two years of age.

For women suffering from birth trauma who have problems bonding with their baby, there are two other factors that may lessen the impact on the baby. One factor is that, very often, even women who haven't formed a close attachment with their babies still make a good job of tending to their babies' needs. Dr Susan Ayers says that it's common for women suffering from birth trauma to do the job of looking after the baby perfectly well, even when they don't feel close to the baby:

> 'I think we need to give women credit, because even in cases where women felt rejecting towards the baby, most of the women we spoke to were hyper-aware of it, and they made a real effort to overcome it. Even if they felt they were going through the motions, they were making sure that they cared for their baby and did what they were supposed to be doing. It's just the emotions that were missing.'

This matches Michelle's experience:

> 'Looking back I think I acted the part of a mother for a year plus. I found it really hard being a parent and I think in some ways I wasn't prepared enough for the change, in common with many other parents. I also think that I was trying to deal with what happened, and that just made it really hard, and I remember writing a diary about it. I kept the diary for about four years, of just little things that would happen, like "She's started walking today", and that was me playacting the part of perfect mum. I was trying to keep this lovely diary, and I remember writing it and feeling really negative but trying to write positively just in case one day she ever read it. And now she's eight, she's a little

poppet and I adore her, but it's taken a heck of a long time, and with my son, I was, like, "So this is why people have babies!"'

Dr Barrett says that this attitude of continuing as normal can be helpful. Discussing studies of children who have survived traumatic situations such as war with their parents, she says:

'The children that seem to be more resilient are the ones who have parents who can carry on calmly. Parents might think that because they're carrying on and living a lie they're making things worse, but in fact that might be the thing that helps them and the child get through in the end.'

The second reason that early bonding difficulties may not have a lasting impact is that when women suffer from birth trauma, fathers (or partners) sometimes step in and make more effort. This is something that Dr Ayers noticed in her research:

'It's never straightforward with family dynamics, because quite often the husband would say, "I could see that's what's happening so I made a real effort, to compensate," so the husbands would often make up for that lack of relationship between the mum and baby, at least in the early months.'

What this means is that the mother-baby relationship, although important, isn't everything. Newborn babies are born into a network of relationships, not just with parents, but with grand-parents, siblings and sometimes childminders or nursery staff. For this reason, Dr Barrett is wary about claims that early difficulties in mother-child bonding have a long-term impact:

'You really do need to take into account the other influ-ences in the child's life, and quite often there are things around that compensate for things that have gone wrong between the mother and child, or if not compensate, then complicate.'

At the moment, there is no research that conclusively proves that a lack of early bonding has, or doesn't have, a long-term detrimental impact on the child. In their study into the impact of birth trauma on couples, Nicholls and Ayers say that, for the reasons given above – many women do a good job of carrying out the mother role, and male partners often step in and compensate for their partners' emotional distance – it is 'not clear whether there is likely to be any impact of postnatal PTSD on child development.'[12]

It feels like an unsatisfying conclusion, but there is a lot more research to be done before we can say with any certainty what the long-term impact of a mother's birth trauma on her child might be.

Learning to bond

If you don't bond instantly, it may be something that will happen in a few weeks or months. But you may want to try to help the bonding process along – no mother wants to feel distant from her own baby. According to Dr Helps:

'Some of the best things you can do to promote a positive attachment and bonding process are: to be close to your baby, to look at your baby, to talk at your baby, and to have lots of physical contact with your baby.'[13]

So one thing you can try is to have lots of physical contact with your baby – kangaroo care, in which mothers hold babies close to their bare skin, has found to be very helpful for premature babies, though we don't know yet how well it works for older babies. It may help to cuddle and hug your baby, or to carry him in a sling.

If you're well enough to go out, you may find baby massage classes helpful. Baby massage is very gentle, and can be relaxing for both you and your baby. One study of mothers with PND found that it both improved the relationship between the mothers and their babies, helping the mothers feel less depressed.[14] There is a good chance a class will be available in your area and baby massage classes run by children's centres tend to be considerably cheaper than the private ones.

You may find similar benefit from attending a mother-and-baby yoga class. These are increasingly common. Rebecca McCann is a counsellor who, with a colleague, runs a support group called 'Butterflies' for mothers who have suffered from PND or birth trauma. She and her colleague sometimes uses gentle mother-and-baby yoga exercises in the group, which she says help reduce stress, and also provide a more relaxing environment in which mothers can play with their babies.

Another strategy that may help is to make eye contact as often as you can, mimicking your baby's facial expressions (poking your tongue out when he pokes his tongue out, for example) and playing games such as peek-a-boo with your baby.

If your feelings towards the baby are ones of indifference or hostility, then actively trying to bond will feel hard. Seeing a therapist to treat your trauma symptoms will help you eventually to develop a warmer relationship with your baby, as well as reduce some of the feelings of guilt and give you a better understanding of what you've been through.

Even though she did love her daughter from the start, Emma was very ill after giving birth and felt a lot of guilt that she hadn't been able to care for her properly for the first three months of her life. It was seeing a counsellor that helped her to gain some perspective:

'I felt that I'd let my daughter down so much by having this awful birth and for the first three months of her life. My therapist said that when she's a year old, three months will be a small percentage of her life, when she's five it will

47

be an even smaller percentage, and when she's 20, it's not even going to be something that is of any relevance to her. And to see it like that – actually those first three months aren't a massive deal to her, even now I can see that, at the age of 20 months, but at the time it felt so huge that I wasn't there for her really.'

***

Sarah's story

Sarah's waters broke at midnight, when she was 41 weeks pregnant. She phoned the hospital, who told her not to come in until the contractions were regular. Five hours later, she and her husband went for a walk, and then as the contractions were coming every four or five minutes, she phoned the hospital again. They told her that she didn't sound like she was in established labour, and that she shouldn't come in.

Twelve hours later, she and her husband decided that she ought to be checked. After half an hour's wait at the hospital, Sarah was examined and found to be 8cm dilated. She was taken to the delivery room, where she was checked and left there without a midwife. For the next four hours, a midwife came in and carried out occasional checks. At one point she was examined and told she was 10cm dilated. Two hours later, a midwife examined her again, this time telling her that although she was 10cm dilated, she wouldn't be able to push for another hour or two because the baby was back-to-back:

'By this point I was absolutely shattered, and I was in a lot of pain, and I could feel that I wanted to push, but the midwife said, "If you push, your baby is going to be damaged, so I held on for an hour, against the pushing urge."'

Sarah was now exhausted and in pain:

'I just remember screaming a lot and after about an hour I thought, "I can't do this for another hour" so I didn't tell her anything, I just pushed as hard as I could, and then I had my daughter, and I took them all by surprise. The pushing stage was recorded as three minutes, and she just flew out because I'd been holding on for so long and I ended up with a second degree tear.'

Her initial feelings towards the baby were not what she'd expected:

'I read an awful lot of books, and I had this idea that I was going to get this big rush of love and be really bonded with my baby, that it was going to be really exciting. When she was actually born, I was kneeling on my hands and knees against the back of the bed, and they said, "Do you want to turn around and meet your daughter?" and my initial reaction was "No". I saw her as the reason that I'd just gone through all that pain and trauma, and it took me a year and a half before I could look at her with love, before I thought, "Yes, you're lovely."'

The tear was then stitched up, and Sarah was given her new baby to breastfeed. The baby wouldn't feed, however, and the midwives were busy, so they moved her to a postnatal ward. At this point, Sarah had been awake for more than 22 hours. She couldn't sleep, however, because the baby kept screaming, and she sensed the other women in the ward sending 'waves of hate' towards her.

Then the midwives arrived. They just came in and took my daughter away. They said, "Just go to sleep, we'll deal with your daughter", and when she came back, she'd had a bath, and they'd obviously given her some formula and she didn't feel like my baby any more. She didn't smell right, she didn't look quite right.'

While in hospital, there was little chance that she was going to bond with the baby:

'My husband didn't come in until 9am, by which point I was absolutely shattered, and I didn't know what to do with this baby. I couldn't breastfeed, and the midwives came in and they kept forcing her face in to my breast, and then they walked away. They just grabbed my breast in one hand and squeezed it really hard then took her head and rammed them together, and said, "There you go."'

After one more night, Sarah went home, feeling drained. She kept crying and having flashbacks, but felt she couldn't talk to her GP, who had become a friend during the time she was having antenatal care, about it. She felt resentful of the baby:

'I saw her as the reason I was in pain, and I didn't love her at all for the first year. I did everything I should do, but I didn't connect with her emotionally – I avoided eye contact with her.'

Through using visualisation techniques and breathing exercises Sarah was able to heal herself and her relationship with her daughter improved. The birth trauma hasn't gone away completely but it is fading over time:

'The further away it gets the less I worry. I'm not having a full-scale breakdown every time I think about going to hospital.'

Sarah's recovery was helped by having a very happy experience when she gave birth to her son four years later. She chose to give birth at home and, despite having 19-hour labour, she felt in complete control, had an 'amazing birth' and bonded with her son instantly.

Chapter 3: Partners, family and friends

Couples always find that their relationships undergo a change after a baby arrives – even couples who haven't had a traumatic experience find it difficult. Relationships with parents, in-laws and friends change too. Most people find this a testing time, but it will inevitably be harder if you are suffering from birth trauma.

Your relationships with other people are an important part of your recovery from birth trauma – but they can also make your experience of it worse. Sometimes other people really don't understand why you are feeling this way, and they may tell you to snap out of it, or that you should be grateful that you have a healthy baby. They may assume you have PND. Even health professionals can be unsympathetic, particularly if they feel they or their colleagues are being held at fault for what happened during labour.

These kinds of comments can reinforce the sufferer's feelings of guilt and isolation. As Emma says:

> 'The worst things people would say are, "The main thing is your baby's OK." And although I'd never wish anything on her, and any mother would choose the baby over themselves, that doesn't mean I'm OK with what's happened to me. That doesn't mean that's all right.'

Partners
Partners and husbands respond in a variety of ways to birth trauma: they may be impatient, or unsympathetic, or they may be understanding but impotent to help. Because it is very usual for couples to experience relationship difficulties after a baby is born, it can sometimes be difficult to distinguish between problems caused by birth trauma and problems typically caused by the

impact of having a baby in the house, such as loss of sleep, extra responsibility, money worries and feelings of resentment on the part of the stay-at-home parent.

There are, however, some common themes both among the research literature and among the women I spoke to.

Anger

Many women feel very angry with their partners for not being more supportive during the birth. Rebecca McCann, a counsellor who supports women with PND and birth trauma, mentions one woman who complained that her partner didn't fight her corner. The woman 'told her partner what she wanted, but he didn't fight for her'. And she said, 'Not fighting for me let me down totally, and if you're not fighting for me, who on earth is going to? You're the father of my child, this is your baby.'

Louise, who gave birth in a Spanish hospital, was refused a caesarean, and felt that both her husband and mother (who also attended the birth) could have done more to argue her case.

'I was really angry. Every time we passed the hospital I got really angry, and we had a massive fight when I went to get the baby's hearing checked, I was really roaring at the top of my voice about why he didn't come and do more while I was in labour. I was angry with him for ages. Angry at him, resentful of the baby and completely terrified of getting pregnant again.'

She also realised that this was unfair:

'I just felt that it's not really his fault. He didn't do anything wrong, apart from not being firmer, and he couldn't have been firmer because he'd have been chucked out.'

Like many women, however, Louise found herself unable to talk about her feelings with her husband:

'He still doesn't know. There's not much point in upsetting him. I was visibly angry whenever I went past the hospital, but I don't see the point in making things even worse. He already feels bad enough that I had such a bad time. We are both Catholics and both very bad ones, but he was in the chapel at the hospital – he was really worried about me. I didn't see any point in making him feel worse.'

Sarah also felt angry with her husband for his failure to support her during labour:

'I blamed my husband for not standing up for me. I got really angry with him, because we'd had long discussions about what it meant to be a birth partner, I sent him lots of links and I suspected he hadn't read any of it. When I was in labour I realised he had no idea. It was his first birth too, he had no idea what he was doing. He saw his wife in pain. I can see that now, but at the time, it was, like, "I couldn't cope, why weren't you doing anything about it?" I remember screaming that I wanted an epidural, I wanted to die, I could hear his voice behind me going, "No, she doesn't want an epidural, don't give her one." I remembered that. That stayed in my head. I could hear it over and over again, hear his voice denying me relief from the pain.'

Although many of the trauma symptoms have faded, and Sarah had a much better experience with her second baby, she is still sometimes troubled by memories of what happened first time round:

'My husband thinks I think about it too much. His approach is resolutely practical, he thinks it was something very bad that happened to me, but it's almost seven years – just get over it. He'll listen to me and occasionally I'll cry about it and he'll give me a cuddle, but he's always doing something else at the same time. He wants to give me comfort but he doesn't think the thing I'm crying about is worth my time.'

Sexual problems

One study of six couples where at least one partner had experienced PTSD found that some women avoided having sex with their partners. One said:

'I think when you've been violated to that extent, you just don't want to be touched by anybody ever again. These are the most intimate parts of your body, your most intimate parts of yourself.'[1]

Women may avoid sexual intimacy because they deeply fear getting pregnant again, or because they have suffered physical damage to their sexual parts during childbirth. Because she experienced a third degree tear that left a lot of scar tissue, Emma found it difficult to have sex with her husband for more than a year after giving birth:

'I was still finding intercourse painful, and I thought, "This is going to be my life forever." I said to my husband, "You need to leave, you go and find someone else" and obviously he said "What absolute nonsense". But that's how I felt: you're better off going as that side of my life is over.'

Emma struggled to get the problems caused by the tear treated by the NHS: her GP initially told her that there was nothing wrong, and although she was referred to an obstetrician, there were several delays in receiving treatment. Eventually she saw a private gynaecologist who pointed out that as well as scar tissue, she had suffered muscle wastage from the tearing, cutting and stitching she'd experienced, and referred her to a physiotherapist. It was only then that Emma started to heal physically.

Sexual intimacy can act as a trigger, bringing back memories of the birth. 'Following a traumatic childbirth, very often women struggle with sexual intimacy because when they embark on sexual intimacy they are re-experiencing symptoms relating back to the birth,' says psychologist Dr Antje Horsch.

It also happens that a woman's sense of self-worth has been damaged: she no longer has confidence in herself as a sexual being. One study quotes a woman, Anna, as saying 'I thought he wouldn't, you know, desire me anymore,' but adding that she stayed in the relationship 'because I thought no one else would ever want me.'[2]

Inability to communicate

Sometimes women who have experienced a traumatic childbirth don't want to talk or even think about their experience – this unwillingness to talk is part of the avoidance cluster of symptoms. Other women want to talk repeatedly about the experience, but partners often do not want to listen. As Cheryl Beck puts it:

'Women experiencing PTSD reported that they wanted to talk excessively about their traumatic births, but they quickly discovered that healthcare providers and family members became tired of listening.'[3]

Some women seem to change personality when they are suffering from birth trauma: they become irritable, over-anxious and bad-tempered. Sally realized that her behaviour was alienating her husband:

'My relationship with my husband has really suffered as he has put up with a lot of criticism and obsessing over very minor things from me.'

Some women simply feel that the experience of a traumatic birth has put a distance between them and their partner. One woman quoted in a study by Susan Ayers and colleagues said:

'He loves me more than ever, he just wants to try and make it better, and no matter what he does he just doesn't make it better.'[4]

This inability to communicate can make the experience of birth trauma even more isolating for the woman.

Guilt

Some women feel guilty that a traumatic birth and its aftermath have created a greater burden for their partners. Emma simultaneously felt resentful towards her husband and guilty about the work her physical condition created for him:

'I felt an awful lot of resentment towards my husband, and I felt like nothing had changed for him. In fairness he has been wonderful, and he had his paternity leave for two weeks, and they gave him another two weeks off because physically I couldn't manage looking after a baby. I think I was probably very, very difficult to live with – not that I admit that to him – because when I let him look after her, I felt he has to do that because I'm such a bad mother, I can't cope, so I almost didn't let him and I struggled on. I felt like I lost everything that day, and life hasn't changed for him.'

The father's perspective

For men, watching their partner suffer in childbirth can be a frightening experience:

'I remember lying in bed with David and just giving him a cuddle, and I said, "Can we talk about it?" and he was like, "I don't want to", and I was like, "Can I just ask you what you thought you were watching?" and he said, "Well, I thought I was watching you die".' (Michelle)

Charise's husband, Roly, felt helpless when his wife haemorrhaged after giving birth. He didn't know what was happening, and staff ignored him:

'I felt completely unable to help or support my wife. I was pushed to one side and not informed of anything. After the haemorrhage they pushed me aside and wheeled Charise away to theatre, leaving me in a room covered in my wife's blood, holding my naked baby. No-one came to talk to me, no-one explained anything, no-one came to support me. They put sheets on the floor to soak up the blood and stop them slipping over. They came back into the room and mopped up with me in the room, still no explanation. I overheard one of the nurses on the phone ordering blood for my wife, and I asked them if she was OK. They said she was fine and not to worry. Having had an army background, I know how much blood you can lose before you're a goner and they ordered four packs, which I knew was life or death, but still no explanation.'

Fathers can feel guilt for not having supported their partners adequately. One man who witnessed his wife have two excruciatingly painful episiotomies without anaesthetic (the second was performed because the baby still couldn't be delivered after the first) says:

'I felt responsible, that I had somehow let my wife down. I felt terribly guilty that I had not done more, that perhaps I had made bad decisions or that I hadn't known what to do. I found it difficult to forgive myself for not being able to prevent her pain.' (Brian, quoted on the Birth Trauma Association website)

At a time when most couples are already dealing with the difficult transition to parenthood, seeing one's partner suffering from birth trauma can be particularly hard. Jean Robinson, president of the Alliance for Improvement in Maternity Services (AIMS) says:

'Husbands are so badly affected, because the woman's personality has entirely changed. They are living with a different woman.'

Men may feel that their partner is keeping a deliberate distance from them. The Ayers and Nicholls study, which interviewed both halves of six couples, quotes one woman as saying that she can no longer bear for her husband to touch her. Her husband says:

'She's a lot more standoffish now of me. At times when as a couple you want to be kind of closer, and then that closeness seems to have something stopping it, there's a barrier to being closer that shouldn't be there. So I think she's experienced something that has made her feel that way and kind of can't get past her feelings and the whole experience.'[5]

Men too can suffer from PTSD after seeing their partner give birth. This isn't surprising, as we know that PTSD can be caused by witnessing a traumatic event. It seems to be less common than it is in women who have given birth, though a lack of research makes it difficult to say how often it happens. Brian, quoted above, writes:

'I was having repeated flashbacks to the cutting scene; it would flash in front of my eyes and I would close them and a shiver would run through my body. These persisted frequently for several weeks, and still continued months later.' (Birth Trauma Association website)

There may be a difference – perhaps not surprisingly – in the kinds of emotions experienced by women and men during the birth. Nicholls and Ayers found that men 'reported more feelings of helplessness and shock than women', while women 'reported more fear, confusion, feelings of violation, humiliation, dehumanization and anger'. They believe that this difference may have implications for how PTSD develops, and that perhaps, 'PTSD involving primary emotions such as fear, should be treated differently than PTSD involving secondary emotions, such as anger and shame.'[6]

It can be particularly difficult for men to find help. Unlike women, they will not be in the care of a health professional in the days after the birth, and so problems are unlikely to be spotted. Men also tend to be more reluctant to seek help for mental health problems than women, and they may feel that they don't deserve help because they haven't themselves been through a traumatic experience. Men (or female partners) can seek referral to counselling from a GP, however. If they don't want to see a counsellor, then it is worth seeking help from other sources. Sadly, there are few internet forums on the scale of Mumsnet or Netmums to offer support for fathers, but the Birth Trauma Association has volunteers – fathers who have themselves witnessed a traumatic birth and who are willing to support other fathers or partners who feel the need to talk. Details are available at www.birthtraumaassociation.org.uk/fathers.htm.

Friends and relatives
Because most people are unfamiliar with birth trauma, women often find that close friends and relatives are not particularly sympathetic to their plight. They may assume that you are suffering from depression, or that it's just a case of pulling yourself together. Women get used to hearing the sentence 'the

important thing is that the baby is healthy', as if their own health and wellbeing weren't also important. Some people also seem reluctant to understand just how traumatic a difficult labour and birth can be:

> 'People say, "I had to have a couple of stitches too and doesn't it hurt when they give you the local anaesthetic", and I almost wanted to scream and say, "No, actually, it was a lot worse than that", and it becomes then [an argument about] who had the worst birth, and that's not something that I want to get into either.' (Emma)

The pressure from other people to be a good mother and to do everything the right way can be intense. Bruised and battered after giving birth, Emma struggled to breastfeed:

> 'I kept trying to breastfeed, and in the end I'd had this brave face on for three days and I'd had no sleep, and I burst into tears in the corridor and a midwife sat down with me and said to me, "Make a decision" and I said, "I'll put her on a bottle" and it was a relief, but I beat myself up for a very long time about it, a really long time.'

Instead of getting sympathy from other people, Emma felt she was judged:

> 'What doesn't help is the assumption not just from health professionals but from other women that you'll breastfeed, and they still say now, "How long did you breastfeed your daughter for?" and now I'm quite happy to say, "Oh, I didn't". And I don't go into detail because I didn't and it's not a crime. But I felt I had to justify it to everyone. I had shingles when my daughter was three months old and I remember the nurse I saw in the doctor's surgery saying, "Oh, because you didn't breastfeed, you're probably going to give your daughter chicken pox".'

Cheryl Beck writes of women in her research study that birth trauma 'choked off three lifelines to the world of motherhood: the woman's infant, the supporting circle of other mothers, and hopes for any additional children.'[7]

While most new mothers seek out the company of other new mothers, through postnatal groups or playgroups, women who have experienced birth trauma often actively avoid seeing other mothers or new babies because it reminds them of their own experience. Beck cites one mother who asked the nurse to schedule her baby's checkups 15 minutes before the clinic opened so she would not have to see any other mothers.[8]

It's a double whammy: women suffering from birth trauma are even more in need of emotional support than other new mothers, but they are less likely to get it. Emma is lucky enough to have her mother living nearby, but even so, the only person she has ever really confided her feelings to is her counsellor. She has stayed away from other mothers:

> 'I'd see friends have babies and a week later they're pushing them around Tesco's. And I think it was six weeks before I properly left the house, because I [physically] couldn't, but I also felt I needed to hide because I couldn't cope, and people were going to find out I couldn't cope and I couldn't do this.'

Sally found that her experience created a distance between her and her friends:

> 'I have told a few friends about what has happened and it has made me feel sad in some ways that their experiences (the ones with children) have obviously been so different. I have tried to be honest about it in case it helps someone else but it's a hard thing to introduce into casual conversation so I do cover it up quite a lot. That puts a strain on lots of situations as I feel a lot of distance from normal life.'

Roly acutely felt the lack of support networks. Self-employed, he took three months off work to look after his wife, Charise, and their children:

> 'We actually lost our house because we got behind on the rent. The landlord was so unhelpful and uncaring, he gave us an eviction notice rather than letting us catch up with the rent. I would have liked some emotional and practical support once we came home – our lives had been turned upside down and everyone was trying to forget it had happened and move on. We couldn't do that.'

Miriam, who suffered an abrupted placenta, and whose baby was later diagnosed first with chronic lung disease and then with Down's Syndrome, was unusual in finding that her relationship with her husband became stronger:

> 'It's thrown us together a lot more, and this is a good thing. We are hewn from the same rock! We're each other's main support because we don't have a close network of friends and family locally. We've always talked, so we do tend to get into quite intense discussions together which plays to our strengths – as long as we also try to remember that there are times when we just need to go and do our own thing that's frivolous and fun.'

Her experience with family, however, was different. They did their best to be supportive from the start, but, while good in practical ways, they couldn't talk easily to Miriam about the effects of the experiences she'd been through. She believes that her need may have been too great for the family to cope with, and that older generations can find it harder to understand and accept the psychological effects of a traumatic birth:

> 'When I was having the PTSD symptoms and knocking back the red wine in the evenings, a relative said angrily,

"You need to be careful otherwise all the children will be taken into care", and I thought: that's not going to happen, I'm not having a nervous breakdown here, I'm always able to look after my children functioning very well, coping with a very difficult situation. At the time I was on constant red alert with a baby on oxygen who tended to stop breathing in her sleep. She'd just had a general anaesthetic for an operation on her windpipe and was still in PICU [Padiatric Intensive Care Unit]. I needed a time to relax, to turn down the volume of the stress. This sort of "pull yourself together" attitude really doesn't help. The criticism didn't feel fair, but no-one likes it when you say that.'

Families are not the only source of support, however. Miriam says:

'Our older children go to a church school which has been very understanding and helpful. The staff liaise well with us and with Ruth's medical team. Our church, in particular, has been brilliant.'

She describes her daughter as a 'truth amplifier': people's responses to her are a good indication of what they are really like, of what their different talents and limitations might be:

'Part of the initial trauma was feeling like I'd been co-opted into a club I didn't want to be in. I love Ruth and I know her now, so it feels more real and natural. But you have to keep going on the journey to feel like that. If you baulk at the start like some friends, our journey still goes on. I don't know yet if those people can ever catch up.

'Good friends who I've known for decades and also new friends with related experiences helped me through. Helpful support can come from family, and also those who have less emotional involvement but who know the terrain.'

Tips for friends and relatives: how you can help

If your partner is suffering from PTSD or PND, it's not easy to know what to do. She may seem like a completely different person – over-anxious, or angry, or tearful, or constantly preoccupied. She may seem indifferent to the baby or obsessed with its needs.

The first thing to realise is that birth trauma can't be made to go away through an effort of will – telling someone to focus on the positives or to put it all in the past doesn't work. Symptoms such as flashbacks or nightmares are involuntary – nobody chooses to have them. So the first thing is to understand that if your partner is going to get better, she needs help – ideally from a professional, but also from you and others around her.

Your partner probably isn't in a position to take charge of the situation, so you may need to be the one who does it. Rebecca McCann says:

'As their partner, you've got to be the one who sorts it out, who speaks to the health visitor, or calls someone like me and asks for advice, looks up symptoms, says to their partner, "Are you OK because I'm worried about you", who takes a little bit of control and says, "Something's not quite right here".'

So do encourage her to seek professional help – she may be reluctant to do this herself, and it can often take another person to persuade her that it's necessary.

Some women want to talk through their birth experience over and over again – if your partner wants to do that, encourage her to do so. It may feel as if she's dwelling on the experience, but in reality it is part of what she needs to do to work through it.

Both partners and other relatives may need to step in and help when the woman is feeling overwhelmed by the emotional and practical burden of caring for the baby (this is true for all new mothers, of course). Rebecca says that it's important to do this tactfully without undermining the mother – while it's easy to assume that a woman would like to have a rest while her own mother or mother-in-law looks after the baby, this may not be what she wants at all, particularly if she is very anxious about the baby. Instead, ask her what she wants, Rebecca suggests: 'Maybe she just wants some company. Maybe she does want a bath or to run away and hide for a couple of hours.'

Many new mothers feel lonely, and this can be particularly true for a mother suffering from birth trauma – attending a mother and baby group where other mothers seem to be delighted with their new babies or chat about their wonderful water births may make her feel even more isolated. So it can help to find out about support groups (whether online or in real life) for women suffering from PTSD and encourage your partner to make use of them.

Finally, fathers can often feel bewildered and upset by what has happened – both by the experience of witnessing the birth themselves and by the emotional changes in their partner. While supporting your partner, you may end up neglecting your own emotional needs. You may also find it helps to see a counsellor or even just to chat things through with a good friend.

***

Jon and Nina's story

Jon's wife Nina suffered birth trauma after a harrowing 42-hour labour. Early on in the labour, an insensitive midwife had attempted to perform an internal examination that caused Nina to scream out in pain and ask her to stop, which she refused to do. Later, while she was attached to a monitor, there was a concern that the baby's heart had stopped beating, and a decision was made to attach monitor clips to the baby's scalp. Two midwives had to hold Nina down while the clips were attached. The monitor still showed no heartbeat, and Jon thought the baby had died, though it turned out that the equipment was faulty. Nina was also refused an epidural until two hours before the baby was born and spent much of that time screaming in pain. Jon describes how it felt to watch:

'Nina was in a lot of pain for a long time. Whilst I know this was worse for Nina, at the same time for me it was exhausting. Trying to keep Nina calm was impossible – she wasn't herself. Nina never really uses swear words but was completely delirious with pain and was screaming, shouting and swearing at the nurses and even shouted she hoped the person delaying the anesthetist in theatre would just die. I don't think she remembers this. I need not say this is not the quiet, loving, caring Nina I know.'

Seeing the anxiety of the midwives when they thought the baby (Tess) might have died was terrifying:

'I could see the look in their eyes and how they were talking to each other had changed. Even though they didn't say anything in particular about Tess, I know they thought they had checked everything several times – the sensors, cables and machine – and this clearly wasn't normal. I don't think Nina remembers any of this but must have been slightly aware at the time as I remember her asking many times if Tess was OK. By now I feared the worst. I thought Tess was dead and it took every ounce of strength I had left to turn to Nina and say, "Yes, everything is fine".

Inside I was in turmoil. Things were so bad I remember thinking all I could do was to try to ensure at least Nina survived this. Maybe this was never in doubt and maybe I was overly tired, but I do remember thinking to myself I had lost Tess and what would happen if I lose them both.'

Jon did his best to keep a brave face and keep his feelings hidden from Nina, but it took its toll:

'I consider myself very calm, measured, pretty unflappable and emotionally strong but by the time Tess had been born I was completely drained and felt awful, empty. It had been a nightmare and I was very shaken. I think I cried most of that night after I went home all alone.' When Nina was home, she suffered trauma symptoms that made life difficult for both of them:

'Nina's attitude did change towards me. She was very short-tempered and, frankly, aggressive at times. I cannot begin to tell you how different this was to the Nina of old. Whilst this made things hard and I didn't like the Nina I saw sometimes, I guess I thought it was temporary. I was a bit concerned when Nina got cross with Tess, especially when she would shout at Tess and cry because Tess was hurting her during breastfeeding but I didn't know what to do. I just tried to do what I could to help and kept an eye on things.'

At the time, Jon had started a new job that kept him away from home a lot, and felt quite isolated, but also unable to reach Nina.

'I did wonder if Nina might come at me with a kitchen knife a few times,' he says.

It took a long time for things to improve. Nina was offered counselling, but the first counsellor was unhelpful. A second counsellor, whom she saw a few months later, helped to reduce the emotional power of her birth memories, and she was able to let go of much of her anger. In Nina's words,

'I no longer wish to stab Jon. Things are much better. I lost my sense of humour for a long time, and we're a very affectionate cuddly couple. And I'm a really soft and emotional person. He said for a long time I wasn't like that, I wasn't myself and he felt like he'd lost me, and I think he's quite happy he's got me back, the normal emotional heaving mess that he married.'

Or as Jon puts it:

'I'm just glad she got the counselling she did, as it made a huge difference.'

Chapter 4: Treatment and recovery

Many women who have experienced birth trauma struggle with it alone and never seek professional help. Some women do eventually recover, or at least reach some kind of normality, over time. Others continue to experience trauma symptoms for many years. Professional treatment is available, however, though the type of treatment on offer will vary depending on where you live, and you may have to wait several months before being seen.

This chapter describes in detail the two main therapies recommended for PTSD, but also gives brief descriptions of other treatments that may be helpful. Website addresses where you can find directories of different therapists and counsellors, as well as contact details for debriefing services, are listed in the appendix.

Professional treatment

Your first point of call should be your GP, who will be able to refer you to the appropriate service. However, PTSD or birth trauma cannot be diagnosed until four weeks after the event that triggered it. This is because, although it is very common for people to display PTSD symptoms after a traumatic event, in many cases these disappear within those first four weeks.

Maureen Treadwell, co-founder of the Birth Trauma Association (BTA), says that not all GPs are fully aware of PTSD symptoms:

> 'If women contact us, we strongly urge them to talk to the doctor and make sure the doctor is not diagnosing them as having PND when they haven't got it. You occasionally find that any woman coming to a doctor's surgery with distress is diagnosed as suffering from postnatal depres-

sion, and PND treatments can actually make PTSD worse.'

Maureen recommends taking along the BTA's leaflet to your GP appointment so that they can understand more about the condition. You can find the leaflet, which is available in different languages, on their website at www.birthtraumaassociation.org.uk /publications.htm.

The National Institute for Health and Care Excellence (NICE) makes recommendations to doctors about best practice for treating patients, based on the available evidence. There are only two treatments it recommends for treating PTSD:[1]

♦ Trauma-focused cognitive behavioural therapy (CBT)
♦ Eye movement desensitisation and reprocessing (EMDR)

In practice, some GPs may refer people to a traditional counselling service if CBT or EMDR is not available locally.

You also have the option of going to a private therapist if you can afford it. When you seek professional treatment, it helps to find a specialist who has a good understanding of birth trauma rather than a generalist.

CBT or EMDR – which should I choose?

It's impossible to say whether CBT is better than EMDR, or vice versa, but some therapists are qualified in both techniques, and will be able to work with you to decide which technique to use. Some therapists who practise both say that EMDR provides quicker results than CBT.

Sheila Marston, a therapist qualified to practise both CBT and EMDR, says they are both highly successful in treating PTSD:

'They're both aiming to do the same thing. They're both aiming to desensitise this very sensitive isolated material in your brain that hasn't got processed in the normal way for whatever reason.'

Trauma-focused cognitive behavioural therapy (CBT)

Cognitive behavioural therapy (CBT) is a particular kind of talking therapy in which patients learn to reframe their experiences in a more realistic way. Trauma-focused CBT is a version of this that enables patients to think through their trauma more constructively. The ideal course of treatment consists of weekly sessions for about 8-12 weeks, though it can take longer, depending on the severity of the symptoms.

Trauma-focused CBT came about as the result of work by two academics, Anke Ehlers and David Clark. They developed a model to explain how the symptoms typically experienced after a trauma persist to become PTSD.[2] In this model, the survivor of the trauma perceives the event that happened to them as a current threat. This threat could take the form of a risk in their everyday life (such as believing they are in physical danger) or a highly negative view of themselves. Sufferers often blame themselves for what has happened. Instead of being filed into long-term memory, the terrible experience is relived and re-experienced, contributing to their sense of being under threat now. The strategies the person develops to control the symptoms (such as avoidance or over-protectiveness) in fact exacerbate the symptoms.

Using this model, Ehlers and Clark developed trauma-focused CBT, in which the therapist and patient work together to talk in detail about what happened to her and, while doing so, enable the sufferer to develop more realistic interpretations of her trauma. The approach helps the patient understand what triggers her memories and helps her to develop other ways of reacting to them. It then enables her to change her strategies for coping with symptoms.

Changing the narrative

We can see how the Ehlers-Clark model works in women who have experienced birth trauma. When they remember what happened during their labour and birth, they often tell themselves it's their own fault, and that the trauma could have been avoided if they had done something differently. Midwife Jane Canning says that women often believe that if they had done something differently in pregnancy (such as eaten different foods or lounged less on the sofa) or in labour (such as refuse an epidural), then their birth experience wouldn't have gone wrong. Emma, for example, had hoped for a normal birth:

> 'I felt foolish because I'd been this person who was going to have this fabulous birth and I felt it was all my fault, and that I'd done something wrong, and because I was no good I'd given my baby the worst start ever.'

Another woman, Alice, kept telling herself in her narrative that it was her fault that the birth had gone wrong. She kept trying to tell midwives that she was in advanced labour, but they refused to believe her, insisting that she was in the early stages. She also told them that she was losing blood, which was bright red in colour, but the midwives insisted that it was a show (the pink-brown mucus plug often lost at the beginning of labour), though Alice was sure it wasn't. The consequence was that the midwives finally rushed her to the delivery suite at the point when the baby was ready to be born. Pushing was very quick and uncontrolled, and Alice ended up with a third degree tear. The baby's cord was wrapped around his neck when he was born. Yet despite the poor care, Alice felt she was to blame:

> 'I felt very guilty even though I'd said to them a few times about the bleeding and I wasn't listened to. You get to a point where you can't do any more because you're quite far into the labour. They kept saying it's early labour, and I thought if this is early labour this is awful because if I've

got to go right to the end and this is only the beginning...I felt very guilty that I maybe should have complained more at the time because if anything had gone wrong with the baby, it would have been my fault. I remember about eight weeks afterwards feeling really guilty that he could have been disabled, or brain damaged.'

Trauma-focused CBT is about learning to rewrite the narrative of what happened during birth so that you end up with a fuller, more accurate picture of what happened rather than one that focuses on the things you did wrong (or imagine you did wrong).

During CBT, the patient will tell the therapist their story of what happened to them. Dr Kevin Meares, a clinical psychologist who treats people with PTSD, explains that part of what CBT does is identify 'unhelpful cognitions' such as 'it's my fault':

'If it [the unhelpful cognition] is "It's my fault", then people will look for all the things that fit with this. The narrative that people often come with is quite distorted because it's pulling all the things from their memory that add up to and confirm the idea that they have about themselves.'

During CBT with a trauma patient, the therapist will record the session and ask the patient to listen to it at home. This enables her to hear the story at one remove, as if it had happened to someone else, says Dr Meares:

'You want someone to listen to it and reflect on it. It's almost a standing away and listening to the tapes, and saying, "It's not like it's me speaking, it's someone else, and I can see that if I were in their shoes, it would be really tough and I can understand why they'd feel that way". It's almost developing a compassionate stance at one step removed.'

He says that there's a question that therapists tend to ask CBT patients, which is: 'If someone is sitting in this chair and they told you this story, what would you say to them? Would you agree that they should be to blame?'

Working with hotspots
In trauma-focused CBT, patients learn to complete the narrative. It's about looking for the 'hotspots': those moments that tend to appear in flashbacks, which are usually the pictures of what happened just before the worst moment – not, for example, the point when the mother realises the baby isn't breathing, but the look on the doctor's face just before that. Dr Meares says that it's as if trauma patients 'have got a hand torch in a dark room and focused it in one particular area. CBT is about turning the light on so they can see the whole picture.'

Clinical psychologist Dr Antje Horsch explains how CBT therapists work with hotspots:

> 'First of all, we have to identify the hotspots of the traumatic childbirth experience, which were the peak moments of distress the woman experienced; these often recur in the form of flashbacks or intrusive memories or nightmares. What we then do is detective work to try and tease out what happened during those hotspots, what were the emotions that people felt. It's usually more than one emotion, it's a whole array of emotions per hotspot, so someone might have been very frightened but also very angry at the same time but also sad. Then we try to find out, what was the particular meaning of this particular moment in time and once we've tapped into the meaning, we then understand those emotions.'

Dr Horsch gives an example:

> 'A woman is told that her baby's heartbeat is weakening and she suddenly feels very frightened and the meaning is

he is going to die, so what we now need to do in trauma-focused CBT is find a way of changing the meaning of the hotspot (given the baby didn't die but is alive and well). When we've found a way to change the meaning, we can also change the emotion and the actual hotspot will no longer come up as a re-experiencing symptom.'

To change the meaning, the therapist may use imagery with the woman, or discussion, or questioning. When the therapist and patient have worked together to change the meaning of the hotspot, they have to insert the new meaning into the memory, says Dr Horsch:

'So we then relive the hotspot and we ask them to say out loud the new meaning, the new appraisal and we then link that up with the new emotion, so I will say things like, "So what do you now know happened?" "I thought that he was going to die." "How did you feel?" "I felt afraid." And then I will say, "What do you know now that you need to say to yourself?" She'll say, "I know he didn't die," and it's important to link that up with the new emotion and to say, "How does that make you feel?" "I feel really relieved."'

This process is about matching up the meaning with the reality. A woman might refer to a point in the labour when she realises that her life as she imagined it was over, and the future she had imagined with her baby and family wasn't going to happen, says Dr Meares:

'The interesting thing that happens is that a woman is speaking to you maybe two years later with a bouncing toddler on her lap, and the toddler is clearly alive, healthy and well, but the memory of the idea of the loss is still alive and well as well. And so we've got this odd experience in PTSD whereby even with clear evidence, i.e. the baby's here, happy and thriving, there is still part of the memory that needs to be gone back to and updated. The two parts of their experience need to be brought together to resolve this difference.'

The therapist helps the patient to learn to 'splice' the new information into the memory. So the memory of 'I think my baby's dying' becomes 'I thought my baby was dying, but I now know that he's happy and bouncing and keeping me up at night and he's alive.'

The patient learns to shuttle forwards and backwards in time between then and now, says Dr Meares:

'One of the things that women will have reported is the idea that it's happening all over again now, and what we want to do is recognise what triggered off that flight into the past and get them to discriminate between then and now.'

CBT in practice
Violeta had six sessions of ordinary counselling, but found they didn't help. She then saw a CBT practitioner:

'CBT has helped immensely. My relationship with my child is great, and it is improving with my partner. I no longer have flashbacks, but some of the other symptoms still recur sometimes.'

Miriam was referred to a CBT therapist by her GP, and the experience helped her to reframe the traumatic experiences of her son's birth:

'I still remember all those things as an awful time but they don't make me want to run around screaming any more. So the counselling definitely helped. I'm not sure if the type [of therapy] makes any difference, but somehow processing events into normal memory – they might be horrible memories – but they don't feel as much in the here and now, they are memories rather than continuing experiences.'

Miriam acknowledges, however, that it is not an easy process:

'I think it's quite a brave thing to do because it does involve going back over all those awful things that happened when it's more human to want to forget about them. But it's actually avoiding it that doesn't help.'

Eye movement desensitisation and reprocessing (EMDR)

EMDR, which was developed by an American psychologist named Francine Shapiro, is an unusual form of therapy that was once controversial.[3] Its use in treating PTSD is supported by research evidence, however, and many trauma sufferers find it highly effective.

In 1987, Dr Shapiro discovered by chance that moving her eyes back and forth reduced the impact of certain disturbing thoughts she'd been having. She went on to test out the technique on volunteers and found it successful. Since then, the technique has slowly gained acceptance and entered the mainstream.

The therapy takes as its starting point the idea that, when someone suffers a traumatic experience, their mind doesn't process it properly. Normally when something bad happens, we are able to store it in our long-term memory so that it doesn't bother us. When someone is suffering from PTSD, however, it's as if the event hasn't been properly stored: we're reliving it over and over again. The aim of EMDR is to help the patient process the event properly so that it is stored with other long-term memories. Dr Shapiro has suggested that the effect of EMDR is a bit like rapid eye movement (REM) sleep, which occurs when we are dreaming. When we dream, the brain processes our memories and stops us reliving them every day. EMDR, Dr Shapiro believes, may work the same way.

Patients normally require between 8-12 sessions of EMDR, though this varies from patient to patient. There are eight phases to EMDR treatment, some of which overlap.

Phase 1 History taking
The patient and therapist work together to identify the disturbing feelings, memories and beliefs that need to be dealt with.

Phase 2 Preparation
The therapist teaches the patient some techniques to deal with emotional disturbance, which the patient can use between sessions. These could be breathing exercises, for example, or the ability to visualise a safe place in the patient's mind.

Phase 3 Assessment
In the assessment phase, the patient identifies the worst part of the trauma, and the patient and therapist work together to decide which negative thoughts to target. It might be a feeling of being in danger, for example, or of feeling worthless because of the way the birth has gone wrong.

Phase 4 Desensitization
This is the key part of the process. The patient identifies a particularly vivid image that represents the trauma (perhaps a look on a midwife's face, or the memory of being held down in labour). While the patient is focusing on the image, the therapist asks her to do one of the following:

♦ Follow a moving object, such as a finger or a lightbar, with her eyes

♦ Listen to a set of taps and tones through headphones in each ear alternately

♦ Hold onto a 'tapper' in each hand, a little pad that sends a pulse alternately into each hand.

This process takes about 20-30 seconds, and the idea is that the memory moves from the right-hand side of the brain to the left. After one set of eye movements, sounds or pulses, the therapist asks the patient to report on what they saw or felt – maybe a memory or a physical feeling. The patient is asked to focus on this thought and then begins the process again with the eye movements, sounds or pulses. The process is repeated several times until the patient reports that she doesn't feel any emotional distress when she thinks about that particular memory.

This phase may take one session or several sessions.

Phase 5 Installation
The therapist then asks the patient to think of a positive belief (such as 'I'm a valued person') and to ask how true that feels on a scale of one to seven. The patient then focuses on the target memory again, while simultaneously engaging in the eye move-ments (or listening to the tones or feeling the pulse of the tappers). Then the therapist asks again how true the belief feels on a scale of one to seven. After doing this a few times, the patient usually reports more confidence in the positive belief.

Phase 6 Body Scan
The body scan phase happens at the end of every session. The therapist asks the patient to close her eyes and check her body for tightness or discomfort or any sensation that shows she isn't relaxed. Then the patient engages again in the process of follow-ing a lightbar, listening to tones or feeling taps. This relaxes the tense part of the body. 'Once you can get the body completely relaxed, you've got a very good chance that you know that this client is almost there,' says Sheila Marston.

Phase 7 Closure

Every session ends with the closure phase. This is about review-ing what's happened in the session and identifying areas that still need work. The therapist briefs the patient on what to expect between sessions, and may suggest keeping a journal to record any experiences she has during the week.

Phase 8 Re-evaluation

Re-evaluation happens at the beginning of every session. It's when the patient and therapist review what they've done in previous sessions, what progress the patient has made and whether anything has happened in the week that has re-awakened the trauma or may need dealing with in the session.

EMDR in practice

EMDR doesn't work for everyone, but it can be very effective. Sheila Marston says that she has only had one patient in several years of practice for whom it didn't work.

Sally received EMDR treatment for her birth trauma. The effect was dramatic:

> 'One session and I went from physical feelings of panic if strangers next to me mentioned anything to do with birth to being able to have a normal chat with another mother about labour. I was shocked that it worked so well, I could hardly believe it.'

This is how Sally's sessions with her therapist worked:

> 'We would talk like a normal therapy session and, for ex-ample, with the birth she would ask me what the worst bit was. She would ask me what main emotion it raised – for example, shame or fear – and how I felt thinking about it now, where in my body I felt that (for example, sick in my stomach) and how I would rate that on a scale of one to ten. Then she would ask me to think about it using a

phrase, such as "I felt out of control when xyz happened" or "It wasn't my fault" and put on headphones that played fast tones in each ear alternately for a minute or two. Then she would ask me how I was feeling and maybe have another go if more things came up. Then ask me to rate how I felt again and repeat if it wasn't a really low score. She said not to concentrate on the tones, just let it be background noise.'

Sally didn't have high expectations that it would work:

'I am very sceptical that anything can get inside my mind and stop me from being ultra-critical of myself but I figured I would give anything a go as it was better than feeling so wretched and I owed it to my son to try. When she explained it the first time I thought to myself, "Come on how is that going to help!" But once I had the first session I really surprised myself. I had a terror of even listening to other people talk about a birth. I was going to a weekly baby swimming class at the time and before I started the therapy one woman had been talking about a friend about to have a baby – I felt like I wanted to scramble out of the pool and run straight from the building just to get away from hearing it. The following week she was talking about it again and I tensed up expecting the same reaction. I was so surprised to find it wasn't there, I just felt, whatever, a neutral, normal reaction.'

Sally had some more sessions after that:

'When I went back I told the therapist it had worked and we did some more sessions on other things that have happened to me. As it went on I could actually feel myself relaxing as soon as the tones started, perhaps as I started to trust it would work.'

Other options

CBT is widely available on the NHS, but EMDR less so. The EMDR Association currently only has 18 practitioners registered in the UK who accept referrals from the NHS. However, there are also a number of EMDR therapists – people who have completed basic training but who have not been accredited – taking NHS referrals. If you can afford it, you may want to consider paying for treatment.

There may be other options. Your GP may refer you to a more traditional counsellor, who will listen to your birth story and help you understand what has happened to you. In some areas you can access a debriefing service with a midwife, who will listen to your birth story and talk you through what happened. Drug treatments are also available, and can help in some cases. The options are listed below.

Counselling

Although not one of the treatments recommended by NICE, some women find that traditional counselling with a qualified counsellor or psychotherapist can be helpful. It is best to find a counsellor who specialises in psychological problems relating to pregnancy or childbirth.

Emma had a referral from her obstetrician to a birth trauma counsellor, with whom she had three sessions. It had a trans-formative effect:

> 'She was the most absolutely fabulous, lovely woman I have ever met…I think that was the first time, through talking to her, that I actually took on board what had happened and how serious it was. Up until then I thought, "I had to have a few stitches and a blood transfusion, plenty of women have that, so why do I feel so awful?" The biggest thing for me was I felt like I'd lost the first three months of my daughter's life and I'd been utterly incapable of looking after her, I hadn't even been able to walk

down the road because it made me feel so ill and I felt so awful all the time. She just gave me the validation to say No, I was right to feel like this, that was OK, that was normal, and I had every right to feel so awful about everything.'

The counsellor helped Emma to think about her experience differently:

'And she told me things like – I don't know whether medically they're true or not, but certainly it helped me, to believe that they were – that to breastfeed when you've had a birth injury like a third degree tear or you've lost a lot of blood is a very difficult thing both for you and the baby, and in the long-term physically I wouldn't have been able to manage it because of how low my iron was. Just to have somebody saying that this was quite a serious thing, because I don't think anybody really explained to me that what happened to me wasn't something that happened to everybody.'

Emma's counsellor was right to say that blood loss and third degree tearing can inhibit breastfeeding – but none of the other health professionals she had come into contact with had explained this to her.

Nina went to see two counsellors. The first counsellor wasn't helpful, but she decided eventually to try again:

'Eventually I became so tired of carrying my mental box (of anger, fury, guilt, resentment, self-loathing etc) around with me that the weariness and being totally sick and tired of feeling how I did, outweighed the fear of actually facing it head on and tackling it.'

This time she had a much better experience:

'My counsellor was fabulous. I've since learnt she takes a holistic approach, and she'd had PTSD herself, so she specialised in that. Her way of counselling was to listen, and it was just a safe place where you could go and talk about whatever you wanted to talk about. And just being actively heard validates what you went through. When I went I felt very weak, and I had a lot of guilt, and I felt like a terrible mother, and a terrible wife and like a failure because women are meant to have babies and women have much worse things than this happen to them. They have babies die and all sorts and they don't get PTSD so I felt really weak. But going through the counselling, she would say things like, "Giving birth, you've never done it before, you've never experienced it, you don't know how you're going to cope, you can't have an expectation that it's all going to go really well." She allowed me to see it from a different perspective. So it's helped me to cope with my feelings and how I reacted to things.'

Debriefing services

A debriefing service allows you to talk in detail about your trauma to a health professional. The term 'debriefing' can be confusing, because it refers to two separate things. It is usually used to refer to a psychological debriefing, in which you talk through your recent traumatic experience with a psychologist. But it is also used to refer to a medical debriefing, in which medical staff discuss your medical notes with you, so that you can have a better understanding of what happened in labour.

A psychological debriefing shortly after a traumatic event can be counter-productive. It may even make PTSD more likely because the survivor is being forced to relive what happened to them, bringing the memory to the fore. NICE specifically recommends that a single-session debrief should not be offered as routine for people who have suffered a traumatic experience.[3]

The debriefing service now offered by some hospitals is the medical kind. The midwife (or sometimes obstetrician) will have access to your notes and will be able to talk to you about what happened during your labour, and why particular decisions were taken.

It is better to wait at least a month after the birth before accessing a debriefing service. It's also worth checking what kind of debriefing service is offered: ideally you want the consultation to be with a midwife who has been trained to listen sensitively to women's accounts of birth trauma.

In Brighton, the Birth Stories service was set up in 2005 by midwife Jane Cleary and sees about 10 or 12 women a week. Women can self-refer to the service or they can be referred through their community midwife, health visitor or GP. Each woman will have a one-and-a-half hour session with a midwife, who will have read her notes beforehand, to discuss the birth. For a lot of women, that is enough, but the midwife can arrange another session if she thinks it's necessary, or refer the woman to counselling. The service is open to all women, not just those with trauma symptoms. Some women simply feel the need to discuss their birth experience, says Jane Canning, who works at the unit:

'The service was set up mainly to give women a place where they could discuss their birth experience, ask questions and talk through their feelings attached to this. Sometimes they really are struggling to come to terms with events and they need the support and acknowledgement of what's happened.'

In some cases, however, the women do have symptoms such as flashbacks, panic attacks and intense anxiety. Because some sessions are held inside a hospital, even arriving for the initial appointment can be difficult for some women, she says:

'Often coming back to the hospital women will walk in the door and dissolve. Just walking in the door again has been too much.'

As well as giving women a space to tell their story, the Birth Stories midwives are able to help women think about their birth in a different way. Sometimes women will blame themselves for what went wrong:

'It's very humbling listening to women, because you can hear they take so much responsibility, and it's not their fault. I explain to them that birth may be complicated and why these complications can occur. First labours can be long, and that's often to do with position of the baby or efficiency of contractions, and they actually affect each other, and that affects the labour. We explain things using a doll and pelvis, and once women understand it, they often say, "I feel like a burden's been lifted," just knowing that it wasn't their fault.'

Women also sometimes want to provide feedback about the service. The Birth Stories midwives participate in monthly meetings with the senior midwifery management and obstetric team at the hospital where common themes and statistics are presented relating to the women they've seen. This information can contribute to improvements to the service in future. In some cases, if the woman has concerns with her treatment or care the Birth Stories team may refer these concerns through appropriate channels.

One of the reasons Charise's difficult labour was so traumatic was that staff didn't tell her what was happening. A year after giving birth, she was offered a debriefing with a hospital consultant, to enable her to find out exactly what had happened during labour and why:

'I found out so much new information about my son's birth! It's been so cathartic. I am finally feeling ready to move on and put it all in the past. I found out the baby was back-to-back with me throughout labour till the last 10 minutes when he turned. As he did the cord went round his neck and the cord blood was tested and showed that he had stopped getting oxygen, which was why they had to do the forceps and get him out quickly. My placenta was partially embedded into the side of my womb and not all of it came out in one piece, which is why I ended up having to go to theatre, as I was still bleeding and they had to stop it.'

Charise now feels happy with the outcome:

'I have had the answers I needed, and felt so angry that they had not told us anything, but now I know they did deal with the emergency well and neither of us would be here if they hadn't done what they did! They even apologised for the way we were treated and said that they would look at making changes in their system of dealing with partners during an emergency as ours was not the first case that had been bought to their attention.'

Debriefing services will vary from place to place, in terms of how many sessions you may be offered or who conducts the briefing. Unfortunately, birth debriefing services are not yet offered universally.

Drug treatments

There is some debate about whether drug treatments, in the form of antidepressants, are helpful, ineffective or even harmful in treating PTSD.

Although NICE favours CBT and EMDR, it does say that there are situations when drug treatment may be offered, while acknowledging that the evidence base for drug treatments in PTSD is 'very limited'.[4] If a patient prefers not to have CBT or EMDR, then NICE says that health practitioners can consider drug treatments. Paroxetine, a selective serotonin reuptake inhibitor (SSRI) is the drug most commonly used in treating PTSD.

Your GP may also prescribe you antidepressants if you are suffering from postnatal depression (PND) as well as PTSD. The relationship between PTSD and PND isn't straightforward, but it can be the case that if the trauma is treated first, with CBT or EMDR, the depression will lift. Equally, it can be the case that if the depression is treated first with antidepressants, then it becomes easier to treat the trauma. Sheila Marston says:

> 'With some people, their emotional distress is so high that antidepressants do actually make living a little bit more bearable. And therefore when you start treatment [with a therapist], it's quite helpful. Other people seem to find that they just don't help at all or they have adverse side-effects.'

Her view is that antidepressants should be used only in conjunction with therapy:

> 'I think antidepressants with therapy in general can work reasonably well, especially as you're working in therapy towards coming off the anti-depressants. Antidepressants in trauma without therapy may reduce the distress a little for someone but there's nothing to help them get better.'

If your GP prescribes you antidepressants, then you will have to be monitored closely, as they can have adverse side-effects. The mental health charity MIND has produced a good leaflet explaining how antidepressants work and what the side-effects are.[5]

Rewind therapy

Rewind therapy (also known as human givens trauma technique) is a particular form of trauma-focused CBT. It is a relatively new technique, developed by Dr David Muss in 1991, so there is not currently a large body of evidence to support it, and it is not one of the treatments recommended in the NICE guidelines.

Nonetheless, some therapists are enthusiastic about the success of the treatment, and say it works more quickly than either conventional trauma-focused CBT or EMDR. During a session, the therapist will use relaxation techniques to calm the patient and then gradually guide her backwards through the trauma, asking her to imagine that she's watching a DVD being rewound on a television screen. Then the therapist asks the patient to view the trauma as if playing a DVD on fast forward. This process is repeated several times until the patient can think about the trauma without experiencing feelings of horror or distress. Typically, patients do not have to talk very much about the details of their trauma to the therapist.

Rewind therapy is not currently widely available in the UK, but if trials are successful, there is a possibility it may be offered by the NHS.

Emotional freedom therapy (EFT)

As with rewind technique, emotional freedom therapy (EFT) does not yet have a lot of evidence to support it, but it does have many advocates. The patient is asked to remember the trauma and focus on one incident in particular, and allow the feelings she experienced to come to the surface. Then she taps parts of her face and upper body several times in a particular order, and rates on a scale how uncomfortable or distressed she is feeling. The therapist asks her to repeat sentences related to the incident, followed by a statement such as, 'Although I feel frightened, I completely accept myself.' At the same time, she carries on tapping. The upsetting feelings gradually lessen, and the process is repeated for different memories.

Support groups

It is always best, if you can, to get treatment from a qualified practitioner, such as a trauma-focused CBT or EMDR therapist, as they have very high success rates and will help you recover and return to normal life within a few weeks.

Some women do derive benefit, however, from the support of other women who have been through similar experiences, either through a postnatal group or through internet forums. Sites such as Mumsnet and Netmums can be a valuable way of sharing experiences with other mothers. The Birth Trauma Association has a Facebook group where members can get tips and support from others (you need to make a request to join it). All these can help women feel less isolated:

'Going on Mumsnet really helped me. It really helped me to see that it was not my fault, it was the midwife's fault. I posted and people said it's not your fault, this is just something that happened, and I posted my birth story and I thought people were going to concentrate on the bad end bit, but people were, "Wow, you had a back-to-back baby without forceps or Ventouse", and that helped me be a bit more upbeat about those experiences.'(Sarah)

'Joining BTA was a tremendous help – just to know that you're not on your own is a really big help. I find a lot of solace in talking and chatting with the ladies on there [the Birth Trauma Association Facebook page]. There was another lady who lives not too far away from me, and she lives about three miles from me and we plan on meeting up quite soon. She's been through something worse than what I went through. If you can help people, I think you should help people.' (Charise)

'I was offered antidepressants but I refused to take them. I was offered no talking therapy and hand on heart if it

hadn't been for Mumsnet and the like I'd have gone mad.'
(Evie)

Although forums can be extremely helpful for some women, they
may also be distressing if you're still feeling vulnerable:

> 'Netmums has a support board for PTSD and I put a
> really long post on that, and people responded to that, and
> it made me feel a bit better – you're not on your own –
> but then reading some of their stories was just totally up-
> setting, and made me feel these women have had experi-
> ences much worse than me.' (Nina)

It's worth being cautious before you approach general parenting
sites such as Mumsnet and Netmums. These sites are not aimed
in particular at PTSD sufferers (although Mumsnet does have a
dedicated mental health forum), and they attract thousands of
posts a day from people using pseudonyms. While they can be
immensely supportive, sometimes people do post cruel and
hurtful comments – bad enough if you're feeling robust, but
immensely upsetting if you're already feeling vulnerable. A site
such as the BTA's Facebook page, where people post under their
own names and everyone is a birth trauma sufferer, is likely to be
a gentler environment.

If you feel it would help to talk to a woman who has been
through a similar experience, you may be able to access a
befriending service, such as that offered by the Acacia charity in
Birmingham. NCT, the parenting charity, runs a free Shared
Experiences helpline, which will put you in touch with trained
volunteers who have also suffered birth trauma. The contact
number is available in the appendix.

***

Rebecca's story

Rebecca, who suffers from needle phobia, had some PTSD symptoms after the birth of her first child. Having made a partial recovery, she found herself becoming anxious and sleepless again during her second pregnancy. Her GP referred her to a psychologist to help address her needle phobia. This was only partially successful, because she was only allowed six sessions. However, the treatment worked well in other ways:

'The best part of the treatment, however, was having someone to talk with about my fears in relation to the second birth. The psychologist directly addressed the birth trauma in these sessions, by asking me if I would consider revisiting the ward of the first birth and talking with someone about it. Our first task was to get me to even go near the ward. The first time I recognized the corridor I had walked down when in that endless labour, I burst into tears and had a panic attack on the spot. On the second attempt I got to outside the ward and peeked in (all the while practising breathing techniques and relaxation).'

The psychologist also wrote a letter to the head of maternity services, explaining that Rebecca had had a traumatic birth and phobias and this was significantly affecting her current pregnancy, requesting a meeting to discuss it. To Rebecca's surprise, the head of maternity services agreed, and they had what Rebecca describes as an 'incredibly helpful' meeting:

'I felt amazed that someone so senior from maternity services took my experience seriously and listened, as I wept and wept. She also spoke to me very calmly and gently, reading through with me all the previous birth notes and explaining why everything happened the way it happened. It made me see that there was nothing "wrong" in what I did, or they did, it was just that it was massively unpleasant for me personally. She sought to reassure me that, if I did come back to her maternity unit (which I did), that it would be very unlikely I would be labouring for three days with a second, and that I would be able to do it. At this time I perceived myself as an abject failure and a complete mess in relation to giving birth; after this meeting, she gave me a glimmer of confidence. It seemed to me that this meeting (which probably took about an hour) was above and beyond what I would have been likely to have been offered elsewhere. It was also intensely personal; I was not made to feel a trouble, or one of many, or in any way that this was an unreasonable request. She reached out to me, as one mother to another. This level of genuine deeply-felt care is probably not standard.'

Rebecca went on to have a much more enjoyable experience giving birth to her second baby – an experience that effectively wiped out the bad experience of the first birth. As she puts it: 'Until I had to write it down for this book, I hadn't thought about that first sleepless horror film birth for months, if not years.'

Chapter 5: Taking action

If you feel that your birth trauma is the result of poor treatment or neglect, you may want to make a complaint to the hospital where you gave birth. An apology from the hospital, and an acknowledgement that you were badly treated, provides recognition that what happened to you was wrong, and can help you move on. For more serious cases (for example, if you or your child has a birth injury that you believe was the result of medical negligence), you may want to take legal action.

The organisation Action against Medical Accidents (AvMA) provides free advice about medical injuries, and it may be worth consulting them. Their website address, along with that of several other useful websites, is given in the appendix.

Even if you never make a complaint or take legal action, you may want to help change things in other ways – campaigning for an improvement in maternity care at your local hospital, for example. This chapter looks at some of the ways you can do that.

Why make a complaint?
One reason for making a complaint is that it may help you achieve some sense of resolution. You can find out exactly what went wrong during labour and what mistakes were made. You can obtain some reassurance that what happened was not your fault, but the fault of the professionals attending you (if that was the case), or even simple bad luck.

Another important reason to make a complaint is that you may improve things for other women in future. The hospital may change its procedures or speak to the obstetrician or midwife concerned about their practice.

Many women never make a complaint because the combined stress of looking after a new baby and coping with PTSD means they are too tired or unwell to go through the complaints process.

For some women, the process of making a complaint may slow down recovery, because they are constantly being reminded of the birth. As Emma, who did make a complaint, explains:

> 'If you've been through trauma, or you've had even a newborn baby, you haven't got the time to write letters and have people come to your house. You think, "I've survived, I'll just get on with it." People are vulnerable; they may not know how to complain.'

Sometimes health professionals actively discourage you from making a complaint:

> 'When the midwife came round to take my stitches out, I mentioned it [the possibility of complaining], and she got really defensive, and she said, "It's a really busy hospital, that's what you expect, I can mention it if you really, really want to, and you might have to go and speak to some people." And at that point the idea of having to go and tell somebody else about it was just horrible.' (Sarah)

It is entirely up to you whether or not you make a complaint, but don't be influenced by people who have a vested interested in you not complaining.

How do I make a complaint?

The procedure for making a complaint works slightly differently in the four home countries of England, Scotland, Wales and Northern Ireland. You'll notice that all four countries have a time limit on making a complaint, so it makes sense to make the complaint as soon as you can.

England

The time limit on complaints is normally 12 months from the time the event happened.

To begin the process, ask the hospital for a copy of its complaints procedure, which will tell you what to do. Normally this will be to write a letter to the hospital's complaints manager. They will then investigate and respond to you. If you are unhappy at this stage, you can refer your complaint to the parliamentary and health service ombudsman.

If you are worried about how to phrase your complaint, or who to send it to, there are several organisations that can help:

Patient Advice and Liaison Service (PALS)
All hospitals will have officers from the Patient Advice and Liaison Service (PALS), and they can help you make a complaint. They offer confidential advice, support and information on health-related matters to patients, their families and their carers. You can find your local PALS office at www.pals.nhs.uk/officemapsearch.aspx.

Independent Complaints Advocacy Service (ICAS)
This is a national service that supports people who wish to make a complaint about their NHS care or treatment. You can contact your local office through PALS.

Citizens Advice Bureau (CAB)
Local CAB offices are usually good at helping with complaints about the NHS.

Scotland
The time limit for complaints in Scotland is six months from the date of the event. There is discretion to waive the time limit if it would have been particularly hard for you to complain within six months – if you are grieving the loss of your baby, for example.

As in England, begin by asking the hospital for a copy of its complaints procedure. Once you have this, the next stage will normally be to write a letter to the hospital's complaints manager. They will then investigate and respond to you. If you are still unhappy, you can refer your complaint to the Scottish public services ombudsman.

If you want help with your complaint, you can contact the Patient Advice and Support Service (PASS). This is an independent service providing free advice and support to patients and families. The service is provided by the Scottish CAB Service, so to access it, contact your local Citizens Advice Bureau.

Wales

The time limit for making a complaint is one year, though in certain circumstances, that can be extended to three years. You can either raise your concern directly with the practitioner or with your local health board. You can make the complaint by letter, by phone, by email or in person.

There has to be a written acknowledgement of your complaint within two days, and a formal response within 30 days. The investigation has to be concluded within six months, unless there are liability issues, in which case the time limit is one year.

If you want help in making a complaint, you can contact your local Community Health Council (CHC), which is there to support patients. To find information about your local CHC, contact the Board of Community Health Councils on 0845 644 7814.

You can take your case to the public services ombudsman for Wales if you are not happy with the response you receive.

Northern Ireland

The time limit for complaints in Northern Ireland is six months from the date of the event. There is discretion to waive the time limit if it would have been particularly hard for you to complain within six months. Begin by asking the hospital for a copy of the complaints procedure. You can then complain either to the complaints manager or a member of staff who was involved in your treatment.

You can take your case to the Northern Ireland commissioner for complaints (the equivalent of an ombudsman in the other countries) if you are not happy with the response you receive.

If you want help in making a complaint, you can contact the Patient and Client Council, an independent organisation that supports patients. More information is available at www.patientclientcouncil.hscni.net. The Citizens Advice Bureau can also offer help and advice.

What happens when you complain?

Usually, when a complaints manager has received your complaint, you will be invited to a meeting to discuss it. After that meeting, you may then receive an apology and the hospital may also decide to take further action.

Emma made a complaint about the community midwife who had attended her during her pregnancy, looked after her in the early stages of labour, and was then responsible for her care after birth. The midwife had made several mistakes, including failing to recognise the early signs of labour (she insisted that Emma wasn't in labour, and refused to examine her), and then, during labour, transferring her unnecessarily from the birth centre to the hospital, because the baby was apparently experiencing problems. This required Emma to experience a speedy and bumpy ride in an ambulance across country roads, only to be told on arrival at the hospital that the baby was fine. After the baby was born, Emma experienced multiple problems, and at one point her ankles and legs swelled up badly. The midwife laughed, and told her that this was normal and experienced by everyone. (In fact, it can be a sign of very high blood pressure and Emma should have been referred to her GP.)

During the complaints process, Emma, who lives in Wales, was supported by her Community Health Council, who she found very helpful and who were shocked by Emma's experience of poor care.

This is what happened after Emma made the complaint:

'The complaints officer came out, and the first part of the meeting was a bit patronising, and "She [the midwife] thought you were ill, she was only doing what's best". Then when I went into some of the details, like she'd discussed other patients, she hadn't checked my baby's temperature, and she put on my notes that I'd declined a check on my stitches, when she hadn't even asked me, they started to take things a bit more seriously, and I talked to them for about two hours. They said, "What do you want the outcome to be?" and I said, 'Without wanting to ruin anyone's life, I want women where I live to have proper maternity services and to be supported properly".'

The outcome was a four-page letter from the chief executive of the local health board, which included an apology and listed the training the midwife would now be expected to undergo, such as the importance of staying mobile in labour. After that, Emma decided not to take the complaint any further.

Asking to see your notes
Even if you don't make a complaint, you may find it helpful to see your maternity notes so that you have a clear idea of what happened and what decisions were made at each stage. You have the right to request a copy of your notes from the hospital.

You can write to or email the data controller of the medical records department at the hospital. Ask to see both paper and electronic records, your baby's notes and other related documentation, such as laboratory results sheets. If you apply to see your notes within 40 days of giving birth, you will be sent them for free. After that, you will be charged an administration fee of up to £50.

Some women decide not to see their notes on the basis that they don't want to be reminded of their traumatic birth experience. When Nina was in the postnatal ward after giving birth, she started crying. A nurse approached her and asked her what was wrong, and Nina could only say that she found it a bit overwhelming and that she couldn't feel her legs (because of the epidural). The nurse told her to try and get some sleep. Nina had to stay in hospital for three days:

'Later on, I was a bit more with it, I looked in my notes, and this girl had written, when I was crying, because I had just given birth, "Mum crying, can't cope". Which is one of the reasons I'm not requesting to see my hospital notes. If it's going to be full of that kind of thing I don't want to know.'

On the other hand, the notes can provide you with valuable information – and, in some cases, misinformation. Michelle had originally stated on her birth plan that she didn't want to be given Syntometrine (a drug that helps the uterus contract) to help deliver the placenta. During labour, however, she was given a Syntocinon drip to speed up contractions. Normally, a Syntocinon drip is left in until after the baby is born, because it too helps the uterus to contract to deliver the placenta.

Unusually, and for reasons that were never made clear, Michelle was taken off the Syntocinon drip before the baby was born. This means that her uterus was less able to contract by itself and she should have been offered Syntometrine to deliver the placenta. She wasn't offered Syntometrine, and suffered a haemorrhage. When she became pregnant again, she asked to see her notes from the first time round:

'I spoke to the consultant midwife and said I want to go through the notes and find out what happened and why it happened. When I looked through them, the midwife had written that she'd had a conversation with me recommending that I have Syntometrine for the third stage and I'd declined it. But that wasn't true, she hadn't had that conversation. And there was a bit of back covering going on because of what had happened. It hadn't happened, I checked with my husband and my doula, and my doula said, "No, that conversation never happened" and I knew it didn't.'

Taking legal action

Some women choose to bring a claim of clinical negligence (also known as medical negligence) against the medical professional or professionals involved in their case. The procedures for taking legal action against your health provider vary slightly between countries.

England and Wales

To prove clinical negligence, you have to demonstrate two things:

♦ Liability. You have to show that there is a normal and usual procedure that the medical practitioner has departed from, and that the course adopted by the practitioner is one that no ordinarily competent medical practitioner would have taken.

♦ Causation: the harm that resulted would not have occurred if it had not been for the actions of the doctor, midwife or nurse. This is decided on the balance of probability – i.e. the action of the healthcare professional was more than 50% likely to have caused the harm.

Alison Eddy, head of the clinical negligence team at law firm Irwin Mitchell, specialises in birth trauma litigation. She explains that, to prove liability, you have to show that there has been a breach of the duty of care that the health professional has to their patients:

'Doctors are judged by medically acceptable standards so we have to show that the treatment that's been received wouldn't be supported by a reasonable group of appropriately qualified clinicians. And then we have to show on a balance of probability that that's actually what's caused the injury.'

Most clinical negligence cases relating to birth either involve cases where the woman has suffered physical injury, or the baby has died or been born with a disability, as a result of mistakes made during labour. In the case of the woman, for example, it might be that a fourth degree tear has been inadequately repaired, leading to a rectovaginal fistula, in which there is an opening between the vagina and the rectum, causing faecal incontinence.

The most common cases involving babies are those where the baby has died, or has cerebral palsy as the result of being deprived of oxygen at birth, or has Erb's palsy as a result of the obstetrician failing to deliver the baby correctly in a case of shoulder dystocia (where the baby's shoulder becomes stuck in the birth canal on the way out).

Alison Eddy says that in the case of perineal damage (such as a rectovaginal fistula) to the mother, there is often a good chance of winning the case although each case is decided on its own facts. Cases involving babies can be more complicated. Cerebral palsy, for example, is the result of something going wrong in labour in only about one of 10 cases, so you have to prove that it was the result of an error at the time of birth rather than down to genetics, for example, or infection in pregnancy. Independent doctors will have to review the evidence to determine what caused the cerebral palsy.

How to sue

Begin by approaching a lawyer who specialises in birth injury litigation. (A list is available in the appendix.) Normally the time limit for clinical negligence is three years, so if you are claiming for a birth injury to yourself, or if you are claiming because your baby has died, you will need to make the complaint within three years of giving birth. If you are claiming on behalf of your child, for an injury they suffered at birth, you can claim at any point until the child is 21. If your baby has suffered brain damage so that they do not have mental capacity, there is no time limit on bringing a claim – though the longer you leave it, the harder it will be to make a case.

If you have already made a complaint to the hospital, that can be helpful, as there will have been a serious untoward incident report and an investigation in hospital. The report, and witness statements from the doctors and midwives who treated you, can then be made available to the lawyers. It is not necessary to make a complaint beforehand – you can move straight to litigation, although to be eligible for legal aid you will often be expected to have made a complaint.

After you have spoken to the lawyer, they will request your medical notes and records from the hospital and instruct an independent health professional (such as an obstetrician, a midwife or a paediatric neurologist, depending on the nature of the injury) to look at the notes and give their view on what has caused the injury. Sometimes the lawyer will seek an expert opinion from more than one health professional – one to look at liability (whether the medical practitioner was incompetent) and one to look at causation (whether their incompetence caused the injury). If the independent professional believes there is a case to be made, the lawyer will then write a letter of claim to the hospital trust setting out the allegations.

The trust then has four months in which to prepare a defence and respond to the letter of claim. To continue with the case, your lawyer will issue proceedings stating the particulars of the claim and the particulars of the negligence. The hospital trust then responds by issuing a formal defence and any statements to support that defence. Experts on both sides will prepare reports and exchange information, and if there is no resolution by this point, the court will order a meeting of experts to define the areas of disagreement before proceeding to trial.

Litigation is a lengthy process, and it usually takes about two and a half years to resolve liability. It often happens that cases are concluded at a settlement meeting between the lawyers before trial when the defendants will admit responsibility, or partial responsibility, and the case settles out of court. If the defendants don't offer to settle the case goes to court.

Compensation is calculated on the basis of two considerations: the suffering caused by the medical error (compensation for the injury itself, including pain, reduced quality of life or mental anguish); and financial loss (loss of earnings through inability to work, care and equipment, therapies and adapted accommodation, for example).

If you win your court case, the biggest sum you are likely to win for the injury itself is about £260,000. When you see huge awards worth millions of pounds reported in the paper, these are primarily for the care of the injured child – a child with severe cerebral palsy, for example, who will need to be looked after by paid carers, and so the bulk of the award will be given in a yearly sum to pay for care for the rest of the child's life.

Some people are nervous of litigation because they recognise that it is time-consuming. If your child has been left disabled and in need of care, however, it is worth suing so that you can fund the care of your child adequately, particularly after your death.

Funding your case
From April 2013 legal aid is no longer available for clinical negligence cases. The one exception is babies who have neurological damage (this includes both cerebral palsy and Erb's palsy) caused by clinical negligence, either at birth or in the first eight weeks of life.

Some people have legal expense insurance. You may find that it is included in your house insurance or car insurance policy, so it is worth checking. You may also be entitled to free legal advice from your trade union, professional body or motoring organisation.

Most law firms now offer conditional fee agreements ('no win, no fee'), so you only have to pay your solicitor's fees if you win the case. Usually, lawyers working on a 'no win, no fee' basis will only take on cases that they feel have a good chance of winning.

Northern Ireland

Northern Ireland operates under the same legal system as England and Wales, and so the process for making a clinical negligence claim is the same. There are a few differences, however. The main one is funding – there is no provision for no-win, no fee cases. This means that most cases are funded by legal aid, says Valerie Gibson, a director at Robert G Sinclair, a Northern Ireland law firm:

> 'Where there's a claim on behalf of a minor, such as a birth trauma claim on behalf of a baby, the petitioners would apply for legal aid. In terms of just funding the mother, it's not going to be available unless she is on very low income, such as benefits. Legal expenses insurance is available, but it is not as widely available or as cheaply available as it is in England and Wales.'

This means that if you are making a claim on behalf of a baby, you will usually be able to apply for legal aid, as babies don't have their own income. However, if you are making a claim on your own behalf (if you've suffered a physical injury as a result of giving birth), then you will find it much harder to fund your case. You are very unlikely to receive funding for a case based solely on psychological damage, such as PTSD.

The changes limiting the availability of legal aid in clinical negligence cases, which came into force in England and Wales in April 2013, do not apply to Northern Ireland.

There are also some minor procedural differences in the way a clinical negligence claim is conducted. Recently there has been a move to encourage the parties in clinical negligence litigation to resolve the case quickly, without proceeding to a trial. It is too early, however, to assess whether this is happening in practice.

Scotland

Scotland has its own legal system, so, while there are similarities with the process in England and Wales, there are a few differences you need to be aware of, too. As in England and Wales, you have to demonstrate two things:

♦ Liability. You have to show that there is a normal and usual procedure that the medical practitioner has departed from, and that the course adopted by the practitioner is one that no ordinarily competent medical practitioner would have taken.
♦ Causation: the harm that resulted would not have occurred if it had not been for the actions of the doctor, midwife or nurse. This is decided on the balance of probability – i.e. the action of the healthcare professional was more than 50% likely to have caused the harm.

The majority of litigation cases relating to birth come about as the result of death or injury to the baby. Cases involving physical damage to the mother are less common, and cases that concern only psychological damage to the mother (such as PTSD), with no physical injury, are almost unknown.

How to sue

Begin by approaching a solicitor specialising in birth injury litigation. (There are only a small number of these in Scotland, and some names are listed in the appendix.) The time limit for bringing litigation is three years from the date of the negligent act or the date when it was reasonably practicable for you to have known that there may have been negligence. For practical purposes, however, if you are claiming for a birth injury to yourself or for the death of your baby, then you need to make the claim within three years of giving birth.

If you are claiming on behalf of your child, for an injury they suffered at birth, you have to bring it by the time of their 19th birthday.

The solicitor will obtain your medical records, and then ask for an assessment by an independent expert of whether the health professional or professionals in your case have behaved in a way that no competent practitioner would have done (liability), and whether it was their mistake that caused the harm (causation). Sometimes there will be separate reports by two different experts, one looking at the liability, and the other looking at the causation.

Finding an independent expert can take longer in Scotland than in England and Wales, because there are fewer experts, and many may refuse because of a conflict of interest – for example, they went to medical school, or sit on a committee, with the professional against whom you want to make the claim. Bear in mind that the time taken while your solicitor finds an expert and waits for their report will eat into the three-year time limit for making a claim, so the sooner you make the claim, the better.

If the expert writes a report supportive of your case, then you can proceed to litigation. The claim will go to the NHS Central Legal Office (CLO), an organisation that provides legal representation for all the Scottish health boards. From there, it can be a lengthy process.

Even if you feel you have a strong case, it does not necessarily mean you will win it, says Ann Logan, an associate at Edinburgh-based law firm Balfour + Manson, and a specialist in clinical negligence litigation:

> 'With medical negligence you're only as good as your medical experts. And if the defenders obtain supportive reports that point in the completely opposite direction from ours then it becomes very difficult to know where the ultimate decision is going to lie with the court. We have to be able to prove that the defenders' expert reports are not based upon a reasonable or logical basis.'

When you have intimated a claim to the CLO, the defenders (usually the health board for the hospital where you gave birth) may then negotiate to settle out of court. If this doesn't happen, then you will need to lodge your case in court using a writ or summons, depending on which court you proceed in, and the defenders will lodge their defences with the court. Then each side has an eight-week period to adjust their case. In practice, each side can ask for more time, and there are likely to be further eight-week periods for adjusting the case.

Before the case comes to proof (the term used in Scotland for a civil trial), the defenders may decide to take the case to an intermediary stage known as a 'debate'. During a debate, which is heard by a judge, lawyers for both sides debate the legal arguments, but without referring to the facts or evidence. The defenders try to make the case that there are good legal reasons why the case should not proceed to proof. The debate stage isn't always part of the proceedings, however, and the case can be settled out of court at any time.

If the two parties do not reach an agreement during the debate, the case will proceed to proof. This can take a long time. 'From the date when you say you want to go to a proof until you actually have it heard in court can be two years,' says Ann Logan.

There are two levels of civil court in Scotland: the Sheriff Courts and the Court of Session, based in Edinburgh. The vast majority of medical negligence claims will be heard in the Court of Session. In most cases, the claim will be heard by a judge, rather than a judge and a jury.

If the claim is successful, then the amount of damages you can expect to receive depends on the nature of the claim. If the case involves an injury to the child that means the child has to have round-the-clock care, then payouts can be quite high to pay for the cost of the care. You can also put in a claim for the child's loss of future earnings, and this will be calculated according to kind of job the child might have expected to earn if he hadn't suffered the birth injury, compared with the type of job he is likely to be able to do with the injury. Finally, you can claim on your child's behalf for damages for pain, distress and suffering, and for the most severely disabled child, this can be up to £250,000.

Payment to the mother for injuries to her in a negligent birth or obstetric procedure are poorly compensated, and all depends on the extent of the injury, whether temporary or lifelong.

Funding your case

'No win, no fee' arrangements are unusual in Scotland for clinical negligence cases. There are three main options for funding your case:

♦ Legal aid. To qualify for legal aid, you must have less than a certain amount of capital – the upper limit is currently £26,239 and this goes up every year. This is more generous than in England, and most clinical negligence cases that go to court are funded by legal aid.

♦ A pre-existing legal expense insurance policy. As in England and Wales, sometimes the house or car insurance will cover this.

♦ An 'after-the-event' insurance policy. This means that if you believe you have suffered clinical negligence, and your solicitors have had a supportive report from experts, some insurance companies will allow you to take out an insurance policy to fund your case, though the premium is likely to be high.

Campaigning for change

Sometimes labour goes unavoidably wrong. The labour fails to progress, a woman haemorrhages or tears, or the baby gets stuck in the birth canal. Midwives and doctors may need to act quickly to avert a tragedy. For the woman, a difficult birth in which her life, or her baby's life, has been in danger, may lead her to suffer from birth trauma. Miriam, quoted earlier in this book, suffered multiple problems in her pregnancy, including pre-eclampsia, and her labour concluded with a premature delivery and an abrupted placenta. She had two blood transfusions, shortly after which she stopped breathing and was on life support for half an hour. Her baby was born with lung problems and also had Down's Syndrome. Her trauma symptoms were a direct result of a very difficult set of experiences.

Sometimes, however, things go wrong because a midwife or obstetrician has made a mistake. In Alice's case (see page 116), midwives insisted she was in early labour up to the point where she was nearly ready to give birth. As we saw earlier in the chapter, Emma's midwife, visiting her at home, failed to recognise she was in labour at all, and told her she was suffering from gallstones. Later she transferred Emma unnecessarily from the birth centre to the hospital, having told her there was a problem with the baby when there wasn't. After the baby was born, an obstetrician tried to remove her placenta manually without anaesthetic, causing her enormous pain.

In other cases, the problem is not that mistakes are made, but that the labour is difficult and traumatic because the women feels that her wishes are ignored or that she does not receive the support she needs. Nina was refused an epidural, despite hours of pleading for one; Louise was denied a caesarean, and went through a painful 37-hour labour before giving birth to an 11 lb baby.

When women with birth trauma recount their experiences, they often say the same things: they feel they weren't listened to, or they weren't told what was happening. Nina and Louise felt their wishes were ignored; Sally was told by her midwife that she (the midwife) was very concerned about the baby, but that she didn't have time to explain what the problem was. Charise told staff over and over again that she thought something was wrong, but was told not to worry.

Midwives and obstetricians are, by and large, concerned with delivering a healthy baby. It's quite understandable that when an emergency arises and a baby has to be delivered quickly, staff sometimes feel they don't have time to explain to mothers or their partners in detail what is going on. What they may not appreciate is the sheer terror that many women experience at this point, and their conviction that they or their baby are going to

113

die. This conviction plays a key part in the development of birth trauma symptoms later on.

How things need to change

Many women have good experiences of giving birth, and have positive memories of the way they were treated by health professionals. There are thousands of midwives doing an excellent job, under stressful and demanding conditions. Evie, whose baby's arrival was a complete surprise, was very happy with the way she was looked after:

> 'I was taken to hospital, given my own room and I can honestly say that they couldn't have treated me better. The hospital staff were amazing.'

For many women who develop birth trauma, however, the quality of care has been a real problem. This can be the result of under-staffing, incompetence, poor internal processes (such as a failure to hand over properly when a shift changes) or simple human error. Solicitors at the law firm Irwin Mitchell have represented many women whose babies were born with cerebral palsy as a result of being oxygen-starved at birth, because midwives had failed to read the traces on a cardiotocography (CTG) monitor correctly. The firm now offers refresher courses for midwives on how to read a CTG monitor – a service that arguably should be provided by the NHS. There are several areas to be addressed:

♦ The recruitment of more midwives. Under-staffing means that midwives are often stressed and overworked, and more liable to make mistakes.
♦ Better training for midwives, particularly after qualification, both in practical skills where needed (such as reading a CTG) and in skills of emotional support.

♦ A greater willingness by hospitals to identify problems (such as inadequate handover processes or health professionals who make repeated mistakes) and deal with them.

♦ Better communication with patients, including a willingness to listen to women's concerns.

♦ Better processes both for identifying women suffering from birth trauma, and for identifying pregnant women who may be at risk of birth trauma.

♦ An understanding of the importance of a woman's mental health.

Midwives and obstetricians regard a healthy baby and a healthy mother as the most desirable outcome, but perhaps forget that it is not just physical health that is important, but mental health. As the British Trauma Association (BTA) website puts it:

'We believe that a traumatised mother is not a "healthy" one and that maternity service providers should understand that childbirth has a psychological outcome as well as a physical one.'[1]

The emotional impact of giving birth can be both intense and long-lasting. For some women, memories of childbirth remain sharp and vivid many years later.[2] Jean Robinson's view is that this is because women's emotions are heightened during childbirth:

'Unkindness, brusqueness or cruelty at this time can go so much deeper, do so much more harm, than at other times. Similarly, the right kind of empathy and support can bring long-term benefit, and many women have told us how a good birth has helped to heal previous damage.'[3]

For most of the women who talked to me for this book, a greater willingness on the part of health professionals to listen to and address their concerns, or to communicate exactly what was happening, or, in some cases, just to offer a sympathetic or kind word, would have made an enormous difference.

What can I do?

If you want to get involved in campaigning for change, consider joining the Maternity Services Liaison Committee (MSLC) at your local hospital trust. The MSLC works to improve the maternity provision at a hospital, and is usually made up of midwives, doctors, representatives of voluntary groups (such as NCT) and mothers who have used the local maternity services. Even if you are not a committee type of person, you can write to your local MSLC with suggestions for improvement in maternity care (though MSLCs do not deal with specific complaints).

You could also consider joining other organisations that campaign for better maternity care, such as the Alliance for Improvement in Maternity Services (AIMS) or NCT, or the Patients Association, which campaigns for improvement in patient care in general.

Finally, you can get in touch with the Birth Trauma Association, a charity that supports women who have experienced birth trauma and campaigns for improved antenatal education, better communication with women during labour, and greater psychological support for women after they have given birth. The organisation's Facebook page is a good way to offer your own support to other women suffering from birth trauma, and the association also welcomes donations to help it carry out its work.

***

Alice's story

Alice's waters broke when she was 36 weeks pregnant. She was admitted to the labour ward at 11pm, but because she wasn't having contractions, so technically wasn't in labour, her husband was sent home.

She started to have mild contractions and lost some bright red blood, which midwives said was a show. They were reluctant to carry out an internal examination because Alice's waters had broken.

After several hours she felt the urge to bear down, but midwives insisted she was still in early labour. She asked if her husband could come in, but they told her she couldn't, as she wasn't yet in the delivery suite. Through the night, Alice laboured alone, and wasn't monitored.

By the morning, she was bent over the bed and unable to talk between contractions. She went into the corridor and tried to get someone's attention, and eventually managed to speak to a midwife just starting her shift at about 8am. She explained that she needed to push, and the midwife took her to the delivery suite and arranged for someone to phone Alice's husband.

By the time she got to the delivery suite she was fully dilated and ready to push:

'They made me get on the bed which I really didn't want to do, but I think they wanted me up on the bed because the whole situation hadn't been managed, so the midwife was just saying, "You've got to push" – there was just no control to the pushing at all.'

The baby was born with the cord around his neck after ten minutes of pushing, and Alice suffered a third degree tear. Her husband arrived half an hour later, while Alice was in theatre having her tear stitched up.

When Alice reflected on the experience afterwards, she realised that the neglect she experienced during labour could have resulted in a very different outcome:

'There are so many things that didn't happen that should have happened, and there could have been very different implications, with the outcome. I couldn't understand why they would keep you in and then not do anything with you, when the whole point of you being in was you're under 37 weeks, but there wasn't very much monitoring apart from when I went in and once at four o'clock, and the cord was around his neck. Now that was OK, but it could *not* have been OK.'

Alice wrote a letter of complaint to the hospital and was invited to meet the antenatal ward manager and the modern matron:

'They had looked into it thoroughly and they did say sorry, and they didn't have a reason why it happened. They said the two midwives on duty just failed to diagnose I was in labour, and missed the whole labour. They were experienced midwives: they had five and 14 years' experience. The ward wasn't busy, the delivery suite wasn't busy, so there was no real excuse as to why it had happened. They did try and say at one point, "Maybe you should have said a few more things," and I said, "I don't know what else I was supposed to say".'

She felt that the hospital had at least taken the complaint seriously:

'They did say sorry and accept it wasn't good enough and they did ring me after to say what had happened with the midwives concerned.'

As a result of the complaint, one of the midwives was put under supervised practice, and the other one had to do a researched essay on the mechanisms of labour. Alice was pleased at the outcome:

'It's more than I was expecting because a lot of people said, "Don't think you'll get an apology because they don't like apologising." But that's all I wanted. I just wanted an apology and an explanation for why it had happened, an honest explanation... I think it's really good to complain, because if I hadn't complained, I would never have been able to move past it. It would have just eaten away at me and I think if I hadn't made that complaint I'd have ended up feeling a lot worse about it all.'

As a result, the hospital were more supportive when it came to Alice's second baby, which she had less than two years after the first. She felt able to express her wishes more clearly, and says the health professionals listened to her concerns. Her husband was allowed to stay throughout her labour, and the birth, though fast, went well. Alice had worried about whether she should return to the same maternity unit, but was glad she did:

'I think it was the right decision to go back there – because it went well, that helped as well.'

Chapter 6: Getting better

Left untreated, birth trauma can affect women for years and years. But with treatment, it can and does get better. It may be a slow, gradual process, but eventually the symptoms can fade and disappear, whether as a result of therapeutic support or through strategies women have developed themselves.

Helping yourself
While CBT, EMDR and other therapies can be very useful in helping women recover from birth trauma, some women develop their own strategies to help them through, either as well as or instead of, more conventional treatments. Sarah, who found herself experiencing some very dark thoughts after the birth of her daughter, has found that visualisation helps:

> 'Distraction, visualisation, breathing exercises, recognising that there's a problem and talking myself round, so when I'm up in the night and I've got intrusive thoughts – I have really realistic images of my children dying, for example, the last one, was my son drowning in a canal, I could see him slip below the surface and I could feel the panic – I just calm myself down and say this is not going to happen, this is a dream, this is a figment of my imagination and I visualise my happy place, and I try to place that one over the top over the bad images in my head.'

For Miriam, whose daughter was born with Down's Syndrome, reading about the experiences of other parents in the same situation helped a lot:

> 'Another thing I did which was really helpful was to read every book I could get my hands on that was autobio-

graphical that parents of children with Down's had written.'

Other women may find that calming techniques such as yoga and meditation may help. Although it is very early days, the preliminary findings of a small study in the US suggests that transcendental meditation can help reduce PTSD symptoms in soldiers returning from combat.[1]

It can be hard to help yourself, especially if you blame yourself for your illness. Learning to let go of the guilt is one of the first steps to recovery. Nina has learnt that guilt is unproductive and says to other women in the same position:

'You are not a bad mother, there is nothing for you to feel guilty about. If your baby is loved and cared for, then you are doing a fantastic job – with your illness you are probably working at least twice as hard as any other "normal" mum just to keep your head above water.'

Having another baby

It's very common for women who have had a traumatic birth to decide that they don't want another child. As Dr Antje Horsch points out, most people who go through traumatic experiences such as car crashes, aren't expected to go through them a second time. Some of the women featured in this book, such as Emma, were adamant that they would not have any more babies. One, Miriam, was advised by doctors not to give birth again.

Making the decision to have another baby can force you to confront your fears head-on. It takes a good deal of bravery and can be a frightening prospect. If you do decide to have another baby, how can you make sure that this time you have a better experience?

It's useful to discuss your options with health professionals beforehand. As we saw in Chapter 4, Rebecca sought help from a psychologist during her second pregnancy, and had a meeting with the head of maternity services, who was able to reassure her that her needs would be dealt with sensitively in her next labour. The important thing is to feel in control of your choices. As Cheryl Beck puts it, writing about the birth trauma sufferers in her study who chose to have another baby:

'Proactive planning and an "ironclad" birth plan helped prepare the PTSD mothers for a second childbirth.'[2]

Research has found that some women who have experienced birth trauma opt for a planned caesarean next time round.[3] The guideline on caesareans from National Institute for Health and Care Excellence (NICE) now says that if a woman wants a planned caesarean because she is anxious about vaginal birth, she should be offered 'referral to a healthcare professional with expertise in providing perinatal mental health support to help her address her anxiety in a supportive manner.'[4]

The guideline goes on to say that if a woman still wants to have a planned caesarean after having had the discussion with a health professional, then the woman should be offered a planned caesarean. The Alliance for Improvement in Maternity Services (AIMS) was consulted on the NICE guideline, and the organisation's president, Jean Robinson, makes their position clear:

'There are women who are wanting caesareans for very good psychiatric and emotional reasons. This is their choice, and it is a valid and appropriate healthcare choice.'

Unfortunately, NICE guidelines are not enforceable. Not all hospitals adhere to the guideline on caesarean section, so you may need to be firm in stating your wishes. It can be worth finding out before you get pregnant what your local hospital's policy is on planned caesareans. Opting for a planned caesarean may enable a woman to avoid a repeat of the traumatic experience of the first delivery and to make sure that this time she is in control as much as is possible.

Louise, who had her baby in Spain, and was refused a caesarean, decided she would only contemplate having another baby if she could be guaranteed a caesarean delivery:

'I've made it very clear to my husband "No caesarean, no baby". I think it's really unfair that everybody has the right whether to have a baby or have a termination, whereas if you decide to have your baby, you don't get the right to do something to make it easier. It seems to be really warped logic to me.'

Louise had her second baby in the UK. The NHS offered her a planned caesarean section as well as regular counselling sessions. She says:

'I found that the perinatal counselling I had in the lead up to the birth helped more than I had hoped – I felt as though I became a far better mother and far more confident just through going to my weekly sessions. I have not even had a day of depression since the birth and was on a total high for the first few weeks.'

Jean Robinson, who has talked to many women who have had traumatic birth experiences, says that, while some women opt for a caesarean section for their next birth, others opt for a home birth. Again, it is your right to have a home birth, but you may have to be very firm in expressing your views to your midwife or GP.

Among the women interviewed for this book, there were three who opted for a home birth the second time round. They felt that staying away from hospital gave them greater control over what happened and helped them avoid an over-medicalised instrumental birth.

Michelle had haemorrhaged after giving birth to her first child, and at the time had felt that it was because the midwife hadn't given her a Syntometrine injection to deliver the placenta. The second time she was determined it would be different:

> 'When I had my son I didn't trust the hospital because of what had happened. I approached an independent midwife and had a home birth with her. That was against medical advice because once you've had one postpartum haemorrhage, you're recommended to be in hospital and have canulas in your hand when you give birth. But I said, "No, I think it's because I didn't have the drug I should have had, and I've got every faith that I'll be able to have the baby at home and everything will be fine." So my independent midwife and I made plans with the hospital: we worked with the hospital, and the consultant midwife at the hospital was the second midwife on call, and we made all these emergency plans, and I had drugs in the fridge. My midwife said, "I want you to have a managed third stage," and I said, "If that's your preference, that's fine."'

In fact, Michelle haemorrhaged again, losing nearly two pints of blood after her son was born, and had to go to hospital. But far from being a traumatic experience, it turned out to be a healing one:

> 'And afterwards, it was like, "Well, maybe I just do that [haemorrhage]". And that helped me to come to terms with my first birth because I'd felt so angry towards this midwife, and yet it happened again with everything happening as it should, so it helped me heal a bit really.'

Sarah, who experienced a second-degree tear when her first baby was born, decided she would have her second baby at home. She had already read books about self-hypnosis the first time around, and was keen to be as relaxed as possible for the second baby. She was determined that this time she would be in control:

'I read books and I taught myself to relax. I read *Birth Reborn* by Michel Odent, and I thought, "Yes, I can do it this time", but it seemed really important that I stay out of hospital. I thought hospital was the reason I didn't have a natural birth the first time round.'

Once again, she had a midwife who she felt was unsupportive – a hospital-based midwife who didn't want to attend a home birth. This time Sarah didn't mind:

'I was able to block her out much more and also I knew I was going to do it by myself.'

The midwife told her not to push, but she listened instead to her own body:

'I lay on the sofa and pushed.'

She called out to the midwife – who was sitting at the dining room table drinking tea – that the head was coming out, and the midwife came in and helped her deliver him. This is how Sarah describes the birth:

'I had an orgasmic birth with my son. All the self-hypnosis just completely worked out, it was a completely painless pushing stage – I had no pain when he crowned, it was an amazing birth. But it was almost as long, 19 hours, he was back-to-back as well, and I had a cervical lip [where the top of the cervix swells, preventing full dilation] but none of that mattered. It was a really lovely birth with him.'

For Rebecca, the good experience the second time round helped wipe the traumatic memories of her first experience:

'The thing that has helped my initial birth trauma the most was a very successful and, if this can be believed, enjoyable second labour. Yes, it hurt, yes, I did shout, yes, it was all a bit messy. But it was simply a million miles away from that first experience. I had intended on a home birth, and started the labour at home, but when my baby was at risk, I had to make a quick blue-light transfer to hospital where I gave birth quickly, with only one midwife in attendance the whole way through. That amazing continuity of care, plus her expertise, e.g. in holding me in a good position when crowning, meant I came away feeling like Super-woman, without a scratch on me, and a baby I could fall in love with immediately. Since then, the good memory has replaced the bad.'

Alice had a similar experience. Her husband had missed the birth of their first baby, and Alice herself had had to go to theatre to have a tear repaired immediately after the birth. The second time round, although it was also a hospital delivery, was very different:

'It was a very fast delivery, very rushed. But it was a very good delivery. The midwife was great, I didn't tear, and it was a much nicer afterwards to be able to have a bath so it was a much better experience.'

This time, Alice's husband was there:

'I cut William's cord and Mark cut Olivia's so that's quite nice. It did help – not make up for it – but it did make it better. It put a little bit of closure on it that I'd had a good experience and I knew what that was like, and Mark was there, that did help a bit.'

New relationships

A good experience next time round often leads to a better relationship with the baby. Michelle had found it difficult to bond with her daughter, but with her son, it was very different:

> 'When I had my son I'd read all about skin-to-skin contact and bonding and attachment, and I just thought, "I'm not letting him go" and I didn't let him go, apart from getting off the settee to get on the stretcher for the ambulance, he stayed naked on me, curled up and feeding and sleeping for 24 hours. I just didn't let him go, and I think that makes a big difference. I felt so guilty about that, and I kept thinking "What if" with Ivy, but at some point you just have to think, "We didn't, and here she is now, and this is what you've got."'

Sarah also found that she bonded much more quickly with her second child:

> '[I bonded] absolutely instantly, I couldn't bear to be apart from him. I carried him in a sling on my chest, and he was always with me or next to me, I wouldn't let my husband take him out of my sight for weeks and weeks. And then at about ten weeks he was diagnosed with colic and reflux and lactose intolerance and he just screamed for the next five months, but I managed to deal much better with that than with my daughter. My daughter was a dream baby, slept and did everything right, but I found her much harder to deal with. I saw her as a thing, whereas I saw him as a person.'

For Sarah, the successful birth of her second child also helped her to repair her relationship with her husband, who had told nurses she didn't want an epidural when she was asking for one:

'It took about a year and a half before I could trust him again, and when I took my son and held him in my arms, he looked at me and said, "Wow, you are completely amazing, I'm so proud of you"' and that overrode the "No, she doesn't want an epidural" in my head.'

Is there a positive side to birth trauma?

When you've been through a traumatic birth, and you're suffering from flashbacks or panic attacks, you're unlikely to welcome people telling you to be positive or to feel thankful that you've got a healthy baby. As time passes, however, and you come out the other side, it is possible to reflect and find good things that have come out of the experience.

Emma, for example, has come to terms with the fact that her daughter will be an only child, but says:

'If I can prevent something similar happening, or help someone else it's happened to, something good has come out of it.'

She decided, two years after her traumatic birth, that she would run in a 10km race to raise money for the Birth Trauma Association:

'Little steps like that for me are something positive coming from something that wasn't positive. There were some things my body didn't do very well but hopefully there are other things my body will do well at.'

Charise found that the experience made her relationship with her husband stronger:

'Having our son has made us both realise exactly how strongly we feel and that there is nothing in the life we cannot get through. It has given me comfort that I know I can rely on my husband. He dropped everything, left work, took over everything – house, kids, cooking, cleaning, washing, looking after me...I think it's given us solidarity and a greater knowledge and understanding of each other. Also we laugh as much as we can every day and appreciate every moment we get to spend together.'

They are now expecting another baby together.

Michelle is now training to be a midwife herself. She was worried about what her reaction might be the first time she witnessed a postpartum haemorrhage, but in fact, she coped well, and her own experience has helped her support other women:

'That was another part of the healing for me, actually seeing someone else go through it. Making sure that they understood what happened and why it happened and just making them feel OK about it was one of my key things, and I could do that and it was fine.'

Nina now works as a volunteer 'befriender' for a charity called Acacia, which offers support to women suffering from PND. She believes that birth trauma and PND can make women and their partners feel very isolated, and that it is important for women who have been through the experience share their experiences. Despite everything that happened to her, she has successfully come out the other side:

'These things happen sometimes to people through no fault of their own – and people react in different ways through no fault of their own. They might have bad feelings, but that's okay – you can feel like this, and get through this and although it might not be okay now, you will be okay in the end. I have become a bit evangelical about the whole thing because I know that it's possible to go from feeling like an abject failure, someone who is

weak and faulty and out-of-control, to feeling like someone who is strong, someone who has come through ad-
versity through sheer determination, a survivor.'

Glossary

Adrenaline   A hormone produced when someone is stressed. It's sometimes known as the 'fight or flight' hormone, because it helps the body take action when in danger by stimulating the heart rate, contracting blood vessels and dilating air passages. Sometimes when women are frightened during labour, their body produces adrenaline, which can have the effect of slowing labour down.

AIMS   Alliance for Improvement in Maternity Services: an organisation that campaigns to improve maternity services.

Arousal   This is another symptom of PTSD. The sufferer feels more alert and anxious than usual, and may find it more difficult to fall asleep.

Attachment   Attachment theory, first put forward by the psychologist John Bowlby, says that a child creates a deep emotional bond with his main caregiver, usually the mother. This is known as an attachment. Advocates of attachment theory believe that a child who isn't given the opportunity to develop an attachment is likely to develop emotional problems.

Birth trauma   The experience of having post-traumatic stress symptoms after giving birth.

Bonding   Bonding refers to the process of mothers and babies forming a strong emotional bond.

BTA   Birth Trauma Association. An organisation that offers support to women who have experienced birth trauma and campaigns to improve awareness and understanding of the condition.

Caesarean section   A method of delivering a baby by making an incision in the abdomen and the uterus. Used in cases where there are reasons (usually medical) for not delivering a baby vaginally. Planned caesareans are planned in advance of labour because a problem has already been identified. Emergency caesareans are carried out when a problem becomes apparent during labour.

CBT   Cognitive behavioural therapy. This is a talking therapy that helps patients overcome unhelpful or distressing ways of thinking. Trauma-focused CBT is a variant of CBT that is used to help people who have experienced trauma.

Cerebral palsy   A condition that causes problems with movement, posture and co-ordination. It occurs because something has interfered with the normal development of the brain, usually during pregnancy. In one in 10 cases, it is caused by problems during birth.

Citizens Advice Bureau   A charity offering free advice to people about legal and financial problems.

Clinical negligence   Also sometimes known as 'medical negligence', this term refers to a situation where a health professional has failed to perform their duties correctly, resulting in injury or death to the patient.

Cortisol   Like adrenaline, cortisol is a hormone produced by the body in response to stress. It can create a quick burst of energy and lower sensitivity to pain. In early pregnancy, cortisol plays a useful role by suppressing the mother's immune system and stopping it from attacking the foetus. If a woman produces too much cortisol during labour, however, this may slow the labour down.

CTG monitor   Cardiotocography monitor. This is a machine that monitors a baby's heart rate and the mother's contractions while a woman is in labour. This is usually done externally, but it can also be done internally, by inserting an electrode through the vagina and onto the baby's scalp. Changes in a baby's heart rate can indicate a problem that may require immediate intervention, such as a caesarean section.

Debriefing This term can either refer to a psychological debriefing, during which someone who has experienced a recent trauma talks through their experience with a psychologist, or a medical debriefing, in which medical staff discuss your medical notes with you.

DSM Diagnostic and Statistical Manual of Mental Disorders. Published by the American Psychiatric Association, this is the handbook used by psychiatrists to diagnose mental disorders, such as PTSD. The fifth edition (DSM-5) was published in 2013.

EFT Emotional Freedom Therapy. This is a therapy for treating PTSD, in which the patient is asked to remember a particular part of the trauma event and to tap her face and upper body as she focuses on the memory.

EMDR Eye movement desensitisation and reprocessing. A therapy used to treat post-traumatic stress disorder, which helps the brain to store traumatic events in long-term memory, instead of short-term memory.

Epidural An anaesthetic injected directly into the spine. It usually offers complete relief from pain.

Episiotomy A cut made to the perineum that makes it easier to deliver the baby. It is stitched up afterwards.

Erb's palsy A paralysis to the arm, usually caused by a mismanaged shoulder dystocia during delivery.

Flashbacks	These are one of the symptoms of PTSD. During a flashback, someone feels as if they are reliving the traumatic event. Victims sometimes re-experience smells and sounds, not just visual images.
Forceps	An instrument used to hold the baby by the head and pull it out if, for example, it is in an awkward position.
Hotspots	Hotspots is a term used by CBT therapists to refer to the moment just before the key traumatic event, and often form the focus of a flashback. This might be the look on the midwife's face, for example, as she realizes something is wrong.
Hyper-vigilance	A common feature of arousal: the sufferer is more vigilant, or more watchful, than usual. For women who experience PTSD after birth, this often takes the form of increased anxiety about the baby.
Independent Complaints Advocacy Service	A free service offering help and advice to people who want to make a complaint about the care they've received from the NHS.
Intrusive imagery	A symptom of PTSD, referring to unwelcome memories of the traumatic event that appear without warning. Whereas flashbacks can include smells and sounds, the person experiencing intrusive imagery has only visual images.
Litigation	The process of taking a legal case to court. The term usually applies to civil cases, such as claims for medical negligence.
MSLC	Maternity Services Liaison Committee. MSLCs are local forums where people who use the maternity service can get together with providers and commissioners of maternity services to de-

sign services that meet the needs of local women.

NCT   A parenting charity (formally known as the National Childbirth Trust) that also campaigns for more choice in maternity provision.

NICE   National Institute for Health and Care Excellence. This is a public sector organisation that develops guidelines for health professionals on the best ways to prevent, diagnose and treat illnesses.

Normal birth   The most commonly used definition of normal birth refers to a vaginal delivery without induction, the use of instruments (such as ventouse or forceps) or general, spinal or epidural anaesthetic before or during delivery.

No win, no fee   An arrangement whereby clients taking legal action only pay their solicitor if they win the case. In England and Wales, no win, no fee arrangements are common in clinical negligence cases.

Oxytocin   This is a hormone that causes the uterus to contract during labour. During breastfeeding, it helps the milk to move into the breast. Oxytocin is also believed to be important in helping mothers bond with their babies.

Patient Advice and Liaison Service   Local organisations that act as a link between patients and NHS staff. It can help you resolve problems you've had with health professionals, or help you make a complaint.

Pethidine   A strong painkilling drug sometimes used in labour.

Placenta   The placenta is an organ that is attached to the lining of the uterus during pregnancy. It passes oxygen and blood to the baby through the umbilical cord. After you have given birth to your baby, you will then deliver the placenta. This is known as the third stage of labour. Normally women are given a Syntometrine injection after the baby is born to help the uterus contract and deliver the placenta. Sometimes the placenta isn't delivered whole, and this can cause a haemorrhage.

PND Postnatal depression. A condition affecting one in 10 mothers, which usually appears when the baby is a few months old. Sufferers feel very low and despondent, and even despairing. Their relationship with the baby and their partner is often badly affected. Over half of women who suffer from PTSD after birth also suffer from PND.

Post-partum haemorrhage This is a severe blood loss (more than 500ml) after giving birth. There are several possible causes, but the main one is the failure of the uterus to contract after the baby is born.

Pre-eclampsia A medical condition in pregnancy (or sometimes after birth) that causes high blood pressure and fluid retention. In severe cases, it is necessary to deliver the baby to stop pre-eclampsia leading to eclampsia, which is a life-threatening condition.

PTSD Post-traumatic stress disorder.

Rewind therapy Also known as human givens trauma technique, this is a variant of a trauma-focused CBT, in which the patient imagines watching her traumatic experience first as if it is being rewound on a television screen, and then as if it is being played on fast forward.

Shell shock This term was initially coined during the First World War and referred to the set of physical and psychological symptoms experienced by many soldiers in the trenches. Most men diagnosed as suffering from shell shock were suffering from what we would now call PTSD.

Shoulder dystocia A complication of birth where the baby's shoulder becomes stuck in the birth canal on the way out. If the baby isn't delivered correctly, this can lead to Erb's palsy.

SSRI Selective serotonin re-uptake inhibitors. These are antidepressant drugs that work by increasing the amount of the hormone serotonin produced in the brain.

Synotocinon A synthetic version of the hormone oxytocin. It is given to women during labour to make their contractions stronger, and therefore speed up their labour.

Syntometrine A drug given as an injection after the baby has been born to help deliver the placenta. It works by stimulating the uterus to contract, and contains two elements: a synthetic version of the hormone oxytocin and ergometrine, a type of medicine.

Ventouse A suction cap placed on top of baby's head. Like forceps, it is used to pull the baby out if, for example, it is in an awkward position.

World Health Organisation The United Nations organisation responsible for developing standards for healthcare and monitoring health trends worldwide.

References

Introduction
1. O'Hagan, E. (2012), 'Can having a baby give you Post Traumatic Stress Disorder?', *Daily Mail*, 23 August. Available from: www.dailymail.co.uk/femail/article-2192214/Can-having-baby-Post-Traumatic-Stress-Disorder-Yes-say-mothers-suffered-flashbacks-nightmares-crippling-depression-.html
2. Bourke, J. (2003), 'Shell Shock during World War One', BBC website. Available from: www.bbc.co.uk/history/worldwars/wwone/shellshock_01.shtml
3. Robinson, J. (2007), 'Post-traumatic stress disorder', *AIMS Journal*, Vol. 19, No 1. Available from: www.aims.org.uk/Journal/Vol19No1/PTSD.htm
4. Robinson, 'Post-traumatic stress disorder'.

Chapter 1
1. Joseph, S. and Bailham, D. (2004), 'Traumatic childbirth: what we know and what we can do', *Midwives*, Vol. 7, No 6.
2. Centre for Maternal and Child Enquiries (2011), 'Saving Mothers' Lives: reviewing maternal deaths to make motherhood safer: 2006–08. The Eighth Report on Confidential Enquiries into Maternal Deaths in the United Kingdom', *BJOG*, 118 (Suppl. 1): 1–203.
3. Full text available at www.dwp.gov.uk/publications/specialist-guides/medical-conditions/a-z-of-medical-conditions/post-traumatic-stress-disorder/icd10-ptsd.shtml
4. Full text available at www.ncbi.nlm.nih.gov/books/NBK83241/
5. Beck, C. (2004), 'Post-Traumatic Stress Disorder Due to Childbirth: The Aftermath', *Nursing Research*, Vol. 53, No 4.
6. Nicholls, K. and Ayers, S. (2007), 'Childbirth-related post-traumatic stress disorder in couples: A qualitative study', *British Journal of Health Psychology*, pp. 491-509.

7. Joseph and Bailham, 'Traumatic childbirth'.

8. Declercq, E. R., Sakala, C., Corry, M. P. and Applebaum, S. (2008), *New mothers speak out: National survey results highlight women's postpartum experiences*, New York, NY: Childbirth Connection.

9. Polachek I.S., Harari L.H., Baum M., Strous R.D. (2012), 'Postpartum Post-Traumatic Stress Disorder symptoms: The Uninvited Birth Companion', *Israeli Medical Association Journal.*

10. Horsch, A. (2009), 'Posttraumatic stress disorder following childbirth and pregnancy loss' in Beinart, H., Kennedy, P. and Llewelyn, S. (eds.), *Clinical Psychology in Practice*, Oxford: Wiley-Blackwell.

11. Ayers, S. (2007), 'Thoughts and Emotions During Traumatic Birth: A Qualitative Study', *Birth*, 34:3, pp. 253-63.

12. American Psychiatric Association, 'Post-traumatic Stress Disorder'. Factsheet available from www.psych.org.

13. Olasov Rothbaum, B., Edna B., Foa, D. S., Riggs, T. M., Walsh, W. (1992), 'A prospective examination of post-traumatic stress disorder in rape victims', *Journal of Traumatic Stress*, Vol. 5, Issue 3, pp. 455–75.

14. NICE (2005), 'Post-traumatic stress disorder (PTSD): The management of PTSD in adults and children in primary and secondary care'. Available from: http://www.nice.org.uk/nicemedia/live/10966/29769/29769.pdf

15. 'When birth is trauma' (blog post), http://midwifethinking.com/2011/05/13/guest-post-when-birth-is-trauma/

16. 'When birth is trauma' (blog-post).

17. Robinson, 'Post Traumatic Stress Disorder'.

Chapter 2

1. Ayers, S. Eagle A. & Waring, H. (2006), 'The effects of childbirth-related post-traumatic stress disorder on women and their relationships: a qualitative study', *Psychology, Health & Medicine*, 11(4), pp. 389-98.

2. Bowlby, J. (2005), *A Secure Base*, London, Routledge.

3. http://teacher.scholastic.com/professional/bruceperry/bonding.htm

4. www.guardian.co.uk/lifeandstyle/interactive/2011/aug/19/bonding-with-new-baby

5. Nicholls and Ayers, 'Childbirth-related post-traumatic stress disorder in couples'.

6. Beck, 'Post-Traumatic Stress Disorder Due to Childbirth'.

7. Beck, C. (2006), 'The Anniversary of Birth Trauma: Failure to Rescue', *Nursing Research*, Nov-Dec; 55(6): 381-90. Available from: /www.nursing-research-editor.com/authors/OMR/16/OMR Manuscript.pdf

8. Nicholls and Ayers, 'Childbirth-related post-traumatic stress disorder in couples'.

9. Gerhardt, S. (2004), *Why love matters: how affection shapes a baby's brain*, Routledge.

10. Murray, L. (2011), 'Maternal Postnatal Depression and the Development of Depression in Offspring Up to 16 Years of Age', *Journal of the American Academy of Child and Adolescent Psychiatry (JAACAP)*, Vol. 50, Issue 5, pp. 460-70.

1.1 Barrett, H. (2006), *Attachment and the perils of parenting*, National Family & Parenting Institute.

12. Nicholls and Ayers, 'Childbirth-related post-traumatic stress disorder in couples'.

13. www.guardian.co.uk/lifeandstyle/interactive/2011/aug/19/bonding-with-new-baby

14. Taniguchi, K., Glover, V., Adams, D., Modi, N., Kumar, R. (2001), 'Infant massage improves mother-infant interaction for mothers with postnatal depression', *J Affect Disord*, 63, pp. 201-07.

Chapter 3

1. Nicholls and Ayers, 'Childbirth-related post-traumatic stress disorder in couples'.

2. Ayers, Eagle and Waring, 'The effects of childbirth-related post-traumatic stress disorder on women and their relationships'.

3. Beck, 'Post-Traumatic Stress Disorder Due to Childbirth'.

4. Ayers, Eagle and Waring, 'The effects of childbirth-related post-traumatic stress disorder on women and their relationships'.

5. Nicholls and Ayers, 'Childbirth-related post-traumatic stress disorder in couples'.
6. Nicholls and Ayers, 'Childbirth-related post-traumatic stress disorder in couples'.
7. Beck, 'Post-Traumatic Stress Disorder Due to Childbirth'.
8. Beck, 'Post-Traumatic Stress Disorder Due to Childbirth'.

Chapter 4
1. NICE, Post-traumatic stress disorder (PTSD).
2. Ehlers, A. and Clark, D.M., (2000), 'A cognitive model of posttraumatic stress disorder', *Behaviour Research and Therapy*, Apr; 38(4): 319-45. Available from http://aidir.home.mruni.eu/wp-content/uploads/2008/11/cognitivehlers_clark_2000.pdf
3. Shapiro, F. and Forest, M. (1998), *EMDR: The breakthrough therapy for overcoming anxiety, stress, and trauma*, Basic Books.
4. NICE, Post-traumatic stress disorder (PTSD).
5. MIND, 'Making sense of antidepressants'. Available at: www.mind.org.uk/help/medical_and_alternative_care/making _sense_of_antidepressants

Chapter 5
1. http://www.birthtraumaassociation.org.uk/policy.htm
2. Simkin P. (1992), 'Just another day in a woman's life? Part II. Nature and consistency of women's long-term memories of their first birth experiences', *Birth* , Vol. 19, pp. 64-8.
3. Robinson, 'Post Traumatic Stress Disorder'.

Chapter 6
1. Rosenthal, J., et al (2011), 'Effects of transcendental meditation (TM) in veterans of Operation Enduring Freedom (OEF) and Operation Iraqi Freedom (OIF) with post-traumatic stress disorder (PTSD): a pilot study', *Military Medicine*, 176: 626-30.
2. Beck, 'Post-Traumatic Stress Disorder Due to Childbirth'.
3. Ryding, E.L. (1993), 'Investigation of 33 women who demanded a caesarean section for personal reasons', Acta Obstetrica et Gynaecologica Scandinavia, 72, 280-5.

4. NICE (2011), Caesarean section, NICE Clinical Guideline 132.

Appendix: Further information

Below are some of the websites and phone numbers of organisations you may be able to turn to for help. The list is for guidance only – it isn't comprehensive, and a listing here does not represent an endorsement.

Websites offering support: for birth trauma sufferers
The Birth Trauma Association.
www.birthtraumaassociation.org.uk

Birth Trauma Association Facebook group.
https://www.facebook.com/groups/52018411070/

A website for birth trauma sufferers in Wales and the UK.
www.birthtraumaptsd.com

Babycentre's Traumatic Birth Support Group, a place to share your experiences and get support from people who have also had a difficult or traumatic birth.
http://community.babycentre.co.uk/groups/a3857275/traumatic
_birth_support_group

Websites offering support: for PND sufferers
A website and forum for sufferers of postnatal depression.
www.pni.org.uk

Acacia, a Birmingham-based befrienders group.
www.acacia.org.uk

A support group for men whose partners have PND.
http://fathersreachingout.com

Websites offering support: for parents

Both Mumsnet and Netmums are forums where parents can discuss mental health issues, including birth trauma and PND. They also have local forums where you can meet other parents online.

www.mumsnet.com

www.netmums.com

For parents of children with cerebral palsy.

www.cpparent.org

For parents of children with Erb's Palsy.

www.erbspalsygroup.co.uk

Phonelines offering support

NCT's Shared experiences helpline: 0300 330 0700

Therapists and counsellors

These are registers where you can find counsellors or psychotherapists who can treat PTSD.

British Association for Counselling and Psychotherapy

www.bacp.co.uk

British Association for Behavioural and Cognitive Psychotherapies.

www.babcp.com/

A register of qualified CBT practitioners.

www.cbtregisteruk.com

A register of qualified EMDR practitioners.

www.emdrassociation.org.uk/site.php/profile/alphabetical

A register of counsellors in the UK.
www.counselling-directory.org.uk.

A list of qualified rewind technique practitioners.
www.davidmuss.co.uk/ukpractitioners/

Debriefing services

Some hospitals run debriefing services for women who have had difficult birth experiences. These are sometimes known as 'Birth Afterthoughts' or 'Birth Reflections' services. The list below is not exhaustive. It is worth checking with your local hospital or hospital trust if it is not listed here.

A Birth Afterthoughts service run by the Rosie Hospital in Cambridge.
www.cuh.org.uk/rosie/services/counselling/birth_afterthoughts _service.html

A Birth Reflections service offered by Newcastle upon Tyne Hospitals.
www.newcastle-hospitals.org.uk/services/maternity-unit_courses-and-events_birth-reflections.aspx

A Birth Afterthoughts service run by Chelsea & Westminster Hospital.
www.chelwest.nhs.uk/services/womens-health-services/maternity-services/birth-afterthoughts

A Birth Afterthoughts service run by the John Radcliffe Hospital in Oxford.
www.oxfordradcliffe.nhs.uk/women/maternity/postnatal/postna tal.aspx

A Birth Stories service run by Brighton and Sussex University Hospital Trust.
www.mypregnancymatters.org.uk/welcome/preparing-for-labour/birth-stories/

A Birth Afterthoughts service run by University Hospital Southampton
www.uhs.nhs.uk/OurServices/Maternityservices/Birthafterthoughts.aspx

A Birth Afterthoughts service offered by Basildon and Thurrock Hospitals. Can also be contaced on on 01268 524 900 ext 3458 or at birthafterthoughts@btuh.nhs.uk.
www.basildonandthurrock.nhs.uk/index.php?option=com_content&view=article&id=101&Itemid=779&limitstart=2

The following hospitals offer birth debriefing services, but currently don't have a website:
Darent Valley Hospital: 01322 428487
Derriford Hospital, Plymouth: 01752 431336
Hampshire Hospitals: 01256 313327

Legal advice
Action against Medical Accidents (an organisation specialising in offering free advice to people who have suffered medical accidents). The website includes a search engine to help you find a solicitor.
www.avma.org.uk

Section of the AVMA website dealing specifically with Scotland.
www.avma.org.uk/data/files/pages/legal_action_claiming_compensation_scotland.pdf

Some of the law firms that specialise in litigation for birth trauma:

England and Wales
Andrews
www.andrewssolicitors.com

Bindmans
www.bindmans.com

Boyes Turner
www.cerebralpalsy-lawyers.co.uk

Henmans Freeth
www.henmansfreeth.co.uk

Hugh James
www.clinicalnegligencewales.net

Irwin Mitchell
www.irwinmitchell.com

JMW
www.jmw.co.uk

Kingsley Napley
www.kingsleynapley.co.uk

Leigh Day
www.leighday.co.uk

Simpson Millar
www.simpsonmillar.co.uk

Mintons
www.mintons.co.uk

Birth trauma

Stewarts Law
www.stewartslaw.com

Scotland
Balfour Manson
www.balfour-manson.co.uk

McKenzies
www.mckenzies-sols.co.uk

Peacock Johnston
www.peacockjohnston.co.uk

Northern Ireland
McShanes
www.mcshaneandco.com

O'Reilly Stewart
www.oreillystewart.com

Robert G Sinclair
www.rgsinclair.co.uk

Campaigns
Action against Medical Accidents
www.avma.org.uk

Alliance for the Improvement of Maternity Services
www.aims.org.uk

National Childbirth Trust
www.nct.org.uk